Marilyn Sawyer Sommers, PhD, RN, FAAN
Lillian S. Brunner Professor of Medical-Surgical Nursing
University of Pennsylvania School of Nursing
Philadelphia, Pennsylvania

Pocket Diseases

Purchase additional copies of this book at your health science
bookstore or directly from F. A. Davis by shopping online at www
.fadavis.com or by calling 800-323-3555 (US) or 800-665-1148 (CAN)

MW01001393

F. A. Davis Company
1915 Arch Street
Philadelphia, PA 19103

www.fadavis.com

Printed in China

Last digit indicates print number: 10 9 8 7 6 5 4 3 2 1

Publisher, Nursing: Joanne Patzek DaCunha, RN, MSN
Director of Content Development: Darlene D. Pedersen
Project Editor: Jamie M. Elfrank
Design and Illustrations Manager: Carolyn O'Brien

Credits

The Nursing Diagnoses are republished from <u>Nursing Diagnoses-Definitions and
Classifications 2009–2011</u>. Copyright © 2009, 2005, 2003, 2001, 1998, 1996, 1994
by NANDA International. Used by arrangement with Wiley-Blackwell Publishing, a
company of John Wiley & Sons, Inc.

As new scientific information becomes available through basic and clinical research,
recommended treatments and drug therapies undergo changes. The author(s) and
publisher have done everything possible to make this book accurate, up to date, and
in accord with accepted standards at the time of publication. The author(s), editors,
and publisher are not responsible for errors or omissions or for consequences from
application of the book, and make no warranty, expressed or implied, in regard to
the contents of the book. Any practice described in this book should be applied by
the reader in accordance with professional standards of care used in regard to the
unique circumstances that may apply in each situation. The reader is advised always
to check product information (package inserts) for changes and new information
regarding dose and contraindications before administering any drug. Caution is
especially urged when using new or infrequently ordered drugs.

Authorization to photocopy items for internal or personal use, or the internal or
personal use of specific clients, is granted by F. A. Davis Company for users regis-
tered with the Copyright Clearance Center (CCC) Transactional Reporting Service,
provided that the fee of $.25 per copy is paid directly to CCC, 222 Rosewood Drive,
Danvers, MA 01923. For those organizations that have been granted a photocopy
license by CCC, a separate system of payment has been arranged. The fee code for
users of the Transactional Reporting Service is: 8036-2234-0/10 0 + $.25.

***NANDA-I does not endorse this usage; please note that a full nursing assessment,
review of patient/family health history, and pertinent diagnostic test results are
necessary to accurately identify nursing diagnoses. NANDA-I stipulates that basing
nursing diagnoses solely on medical diagnoses or conditions can lead to inaccurate
nursing diagnoses, and to inappropriate care.**

List of Reviewers

Contents

Skin   1

Head and Neck   9

Respiratory and Chest   18

Cardiovascular and Peripheral Vascular   51

Gastrointestinal and Hepatobiliary   94

Renal and Urologic   142

Musculoskeletal   174

Neurological   192

Endocrine and Metabolic   231

Hematologic and Immune   263

Acid-Base and Fluid and Electrolyte Imbalances   300

Trauma and Emergency Care   325

Infection   339

Index   349

Burns

Approximately 700,000 visits to emergency departments occur each year because of burns. While most burns are not life threatening, they cause pain and injury. Skin is very fragile; when temperatures reach more than 120°F, skin burns so severely that surgery may be needed.

Burns damage not only the outer parts of the body, such as skin, but can injure internal structures such as muscles, fascia, bone, and nerves. As a result of the number of layers of skin and tissue that are damaged, burns are characterized as first, second, third, or fourth degree. The skin injury from burns has six different mechanisms of injury: scalds, contact burns, fire, chemical, electrical, and radiation.

Where It Occurs

- Preschool children account for over two-thirds of all burn fatalities.
- Serious burn injuries occur most commonly in males, and in particular, young adult males ages 20 to 29 years, followed by children under 9 years.
- Individuals older than 50 years sustain the fewest number of serious burn injuries.

Signal Symptoms

- First-degree burn: erythema, blanching on pressure, mild to moderate pain, no blister (typical of sunburn). Only structure involved is the epidermis.
- Second-degree burn: superficially, the papillary dermis is affected with blisters, redness, and severe pain because of exposed nerve endings; on a deeper level, the reticular dermis is affected with blisters, pale white or yellow color, and an absence of pain sensation.
- Third-degree burn: all levels of the dermis along with subcutaneous fat are affected; blisters may be absent with leathery, wrinkled skin without capillary refill; thrombosed blood vessels are visible; pain insensitivity occurs because of nerve destruction.
- Fourth-degree burn: involves all levels of dermis as well as fascia, muscle, and bone.

Skin

BE SAFE! Basic assessment of airway, breathing, and circulation (ABCs) takes first priority.

Diagnostic Tests

Test	What It Tells	Patient Problems/ Nursing Care
Fiberoptic bronchoscopy	Shows thermal injury and edema to oropharynx and glottis	Knowledge deficit: explain procedures. NPO and sedation and pain control may be necessary.
Carboxyhemoglobin levels	>10% indicates potential inhalation injury; >30% is associated with mental status changes; >60% is lethal	Knowledge deficit: explain procedures. Patient will need venipuncture.

Treatment and Nursing Care

Potential Nursing Diagnoses*

Ineffective airway clearance
Impaired skin integrity
Fluid volume deficit
Hypothermia
Risk for infection

BE SMART! Large burns cause loss of fluid that needs to be replaced with fluid resuscitation. Warm all fluids.

- Silver sulfadiazine, topical antimicrobial agent, is a cream that lowers bacterial counts, minimizes water evaporation, and decreases heat loss.
- Mafenide acetate, another topical antimicrobial agent, provides coverage for gram-negative and anaerobic bacteria; allows for deep eschar penetration.
- Minor burn wounds are cared for by using the principles of comfort, cleanliness, and infection control.

- For patients with a major injury, the course of recovery is divided into four phases: emergent-resuscitative, acute-wound coverage, convalescent-rehabilitative, and reorganization-reintegration.
- The highest priority for the burn patient is to maintain the ABCs.

Cellulitis

Cellulitis is an acute, rapidly spreading infection of the skin and subcutaneous tissues. It is characterized by hyperemia, swelling, and leukocyte infiltration. It is a nonnecrotizing inflammation that does not involve the fascia or muscles.

The infection is caused by bacteria entering the bloodstream via a disruption in the skin integrity, usually after a bite, laceration, abrasion, blister, burn, or puncture wound, or it may be an extension from a contiguous focus, such as an abscess or a metastatic dissemination from bacteremia. Most cases of cellulitis are caused by *Streptococcus pyogenes* or *Staphylococcus aureus*.

Where It Occurs

- Occurs in all ages, ethnicities, and genders.
- Although it can be caused by bites and lacerations or wounds, it can also occur without evidence of injury.
- Associated with people who have systemic diseases such as diabetes mellitus, immunodeficiency, cancer, chronic kidney or liver disease, and peripheral vascular disease.

Signal Symptoms

- Typically a history of trauma followed by local tenderness, pain, warmth, erythema, chills, high fever, malaise, regional lymphadenopathy, and occasionally swelling.
- Progression of symptoms can be rapid.

BE SAFE! Patient needs antibiotics promptly so that the infection does not become systemic and progress to sepsis. If a red streak appears migrating from an area of cellulitis, the infection may be spreading and antibiotics should possibly be changed.

Diagnostic Tests

Test	What It Tells	Patient Problems/ Nursing Care
Blood culture	Determines the type of bacteria, if any, involved in the infection	Knowledge deficit: explain procedures. Patient will need venipuncture.

Treatment and Nursing Care

Potential Nursing Diagnoses*

Risk for infection
Impaired tissue integrity
Pain (acute)

BE SMART! Teach patients to take all the antibiotics until the prescription is finished.

- Most people can be treated on an outpatient basis for cellulitis.
- Activity using the affected extremity may be painful; elevation of the extremity may relieve discomfort.
- Over-the-counter analgesia such as acetaminophen or ibuprofen usually helps relieve pain and discomfort.
- A health-care provider should be notified for fever and chills or increased immobility in the affected extremity.

Herpes Zoster

Herpes zoster, also known as *shingles*, is a common viral skin eruption. It is caused by a reactivation of the varicella zoster virus (VZV), which causes chickenpox. Herpes zoster causes acute unilateral inflammation of a dorsal root ganglion. Each nerve innervates a particular skin area on the body called a *dermatome*, which bends around the body in a pattern that has been mapped corresponding to the vertebral source.

Most patients recover completely, but approximately 12% experience complications that include postherpetic neuralgia (PHN), uveitis, motor deficits, infection, and systemic involvement such as meningoencephalitis, pneumonia, deafness, or widespread dissemination. Shingles often is associated with immunosuppression and occurs in people with cancer, on immunosuppressive drugs, and during times of excessive emotional or physiological stress.

Where It Occurs

- Prevalence doubles in patients over age 50, and approximately 80% of all cases occur in people older than 20 years.
- Herpes zoster can occur at any age and in both genders, although it is uncommon in healthy children and young adults.
- Outbreaks of shingles are associated with immune suppression.

Signal Symptoms

- Itching, numbness, tingling, tenderness, and pain in the affected area for 1 to 2 days before skin lesions develop.
- Rash: maculopapules (discolored patches on the skin mixed with elevated red pimples) that rapidly develop into crops of vesicles (blisters) on an erythematous (diffuse redness) base.
- New lesions continue to appear for 3 to 5 days as the older lesions ulcerate and crust. Malaise, low-grade fever, and adenopathy may accompany the rash.

BE SAFE! Observe the rash, noting the color, temperature, and appearance of lesions and their location and distribution over the body.

Diagnostic Tests

Test	What It Tells	Patient Problems/ Nursing Care
Polymerase chain reaction	Positive result for herpes zoster DNA	Knowledge deficit: explain procedures. Patient will need venipuncture.
Viral culture	Positive result for herpes zoster	Knowledge deficit: explain procedures.

Treatment and Nursing Care

Potential Nursing Diagnoses*

Pain (acute or chronic)
Impaired skin integrity
Risk for infection
Anxiety
Knowledge deficit (skin care, medications)

> **BE SMART!** Shingles vaccine is available from primary care providers and, while expensive, reduces the risk of developing the condition; rates are 55% lower with people who receive the vaccine as compared to those who do not.

- Antivirals are used to treat herpes zoster.
- Topical analgesics, such as capsaicin (Zostrix), are used to treat neuralgia after shingles.
- Antihistamines may help with itching, and topical lidocaine sprays can be used to provide analgesia.
- Monitor patient's levels of pain, which can be excruciating. Pain relief may vary from the use of mild analgesics (e.g., aspirin or acetaminophen) to mild opiates (e.g., codeine) if the pain is severe. The use of systemic corticosteroids appears to decrease the severity of PHN pain.
- Nighttime sedation also may be helpful.
- Teach patient how to manage skin care and about medications.

Pressure Ulcer

A pressure ulcer is an irregularly shaped, depressed area that results from necrosis of the epidermis and/or dermis layers of the skin. Prolonged pressure causes inadequate circulation, ischemic ulceration, and tissue breakdown.

Pressure ulcers may occur in any area of the body but occur mostly over bony prominences. Some 96% of pressure ulcers develop in the lower part of the body, with the common sites including the ischium (28%), the sacrum (18%–27%), the trochanter (12%–20%), and the heel (10%–18%). Pressure ulcers have been staged by the National Ulcer Advisory Panel, but the stages serve as a description only and do not necessarily provide an order for progression.

Where It Occurs

- Pressure ulcers can occur at any age and across both genders but are more prevalent in the elderly population over 70 years of age.
- About 25% of the elderly have some type of pressure ulcer, and most of these individuals are women because of their survival advantage over men.
- Pressure ulcers are also common in individuals who are neurologically impaired, have nutritional or perfusion deficits, and are immobile.

Signal Symptoms

- Stage I: nonblanchable erythema; involves changes in the underlying vessels of the skin; bright red color that does not resolve after 30 minutes of pressure relief; can be painful and tender.
- Stage II: partial-thickness skin loss of epidermis and dermis; cracks or blisters on skin with erythema and/or indurations.
- Stage III: full-thickness skin loss of epidermis and dermis; extends down to subcutaneous tissue; appears as a crater or covered by black eschar; wound base usually not painful; indistinct borders; may have sinus tracts or undermining present.
- Stage IV: full-thickness skin loss with extensive destruction of tissue, muscle, bone, and/or supporting structures; appears as a deep crater or is covered by thick eschar; wound base not painful; may have sinus tracts and undermining present.

BE SAFE! Assess at-risk patients frequently for early signs of skin breakdown at most common sites of occurrence.

Diagnostic Tests

Test	What It Tells	Patient Problems/ Nursing Care
Skin or wound culture and sensitivity	Positive result for microorganisms	Knowledge deficit: explain all procedures.
Braden Scale	Predicts pressure sore risk (score of 15–16 = low risk; 13–14 = moderate risk; 12 or less = high risk)	Knowledge deficit: explain all procedures.

Treatment and Nursing Care

Potential Nursing Diagnoses*

Impaired skin integrity
Ineffective tissue perfusion (peripheral)
Impaired physical mobility
Risk for infection

> **BE SMART!** The high-risk patient needs turning and proper
> positioning at least every 2 hours.

- Hydrocolloids are used as occlusive, adhesive wafers.
- Hydrogels are used to promote healing by rehydrating necrotic tissue.
- The most important nursing intervention is prevention.
- Pressure-relieving devices, such as silicone-filled pads and foam
  mattresses, may be helpful.

Cancer, Oral

Oral cancers include all of those occurring on the lip, tongue, floor of mouth, pharynx, salivary glands, inside of cheeks, gums, and palate. The lower lip is the most common site and has the best prognosis. Ninety percent are squamous cell carcinomas, which may result from immune alterations such as local imbalances in T-cell function and Epstein-Barr virus. Use of tobacco including chewing tobacco or betel leaves, heavy alcohol use, and exposure to ultraviolet light are all contributing factors. Five-year survival rate is more than 70%.

Where It Occurs

- Seventy-five percent of all cases occur in adults over age 60.
- Occurs in men more than in women.
- Often occurs on the lip and lateral portion of the tongue.

Signal Symptoms

- Persistence of a lump or sore within the oral cavity.
- Mild soreness when eating, a lesion or lump in the mouth, problems with articulation.
- Late: pain, weight loss, enlarged cervical lymph nodes, impaired airway.

BE SAFE! Encourage patient to have all lesions that do not heal assessed by a health-care practitioner.

Diagnostic Tests

Test	What It Tells	Patient Problems/ Nursing Care
Liver function tests	A normal result rules out metastasis	Knowledge deficit: explain procedures. Patient will need venipuncture.
Biopsy	Confirms diagnosis of any lesion present for more than 4–6 weeks	Knowledge deficit: explain procedures. Check for bleeding and infection.

Treatment and Nursing Care

Potential Nursing Diagnoses*

Impaired oral mucous membrane
Pain (acute)
Impaired swallowing
Impaired tissue integrity
Disturbed body image

> **BE SMART!** Provide teaching materials to help patients reduce problem drinking or tobacco use.

- Oral squamous cell carcinomas are usually treated surgically and/or with irradiation.
- Oral mucositis occurs with external beam radiotherapy or cancer chemotherapy; it is very distressing and has important negative effects on quality of life.
- Patient education directed at behavioral change for smoking cessation or sensible alcohol use.

Candidiasis, Oral

Oropharyngeal candidiasis is an abnormal overgrowth in the oral cavity of the yeastlike fungus *Candida albicans* or, less commonly, *Candida tropicalis. Candida* species colonize human mucocutaneous surfaces, and most infections are acquired from pre-existing reservoirs in the body when patients have usual physiological stress such as burns, severe trauma, and solid neoplasms.

Candidiasis is readily treatable but often recurs in immunocompromised patients. Mucosal and systemic candidiasis is a growing health problem grounded in the large numbers of patients with immune compromise without protection in tissues normally resistant to invasion.

The increased prevalence of *Candida* infections has led to a range of diseases from superficial mucocutaneous disease to invasive illnesses such as *Candida* peritonitis and systemic infections.

Where It Occurs

- Rare in otherwise healthy adults; typically reflects an underlying immunocompromised state.
- Among immunocompromised patients, candidiasis is most commonly seen in newborns and older patients.

Signal Symptoms

- White, painless, exudative patches with an erythematous base are easily scraped from buccal mucosa, tongue, posterior pharynx.
- Excessive dryness of the mouth, foul breath, sores at the corners of the mouth.

BE SAFE! Repeated candidiasis may indicate that the patient is immunocompromised and may require further investigation by a health-care provider.

Diagnostic Tests

Test	What It Tells	Patient Problems/ Nursing Care
Gram stain or wet mount	Demonstrates budding yeast forms indicating candidal fungal infections	Knowledge deficit: explain procedures.

Treatment and Nursing Care

Potential Nursing Diagnoses*

Impaired oral mucous membrane
Impaired tissue integrity
Impaired swallowing
Imbalanced nutrition, less than body requirements

BE SMART! Beware of fluoride toothpaste sensitivity, especially in patients with dental braces; the angular cheilitis mimics candidiasis.

- Antifungal medications: nystatin, clotrimazole, amphotericin B oral suspension or systemic oral azoles (fluconazole, itraconazole, or posaconazole).
- Note that infections in HIV-positive patients may respond slowly and recur often.
- Assess the underlying immune status.
- Avoid abrasive oral products and encourage a nonirritating diet until the infection is under control.

Epistaxis

Epistaxis, commonly called a *nosebleed*, is a hemorrhage of the nasal mucosa resulting from the traumatic or spontaneous rupture of superficial capillaries, veins, or arteries. Most are benign and self-limiting but in some children can recur. Bleeding occurs when the nasal mucosa is irritated, torn, scraped, or eroded. The blood vessels are exposed and break, allowing for blood flow. Epistaxis may be classified as anterior or posterior, depending on the location of the bleeding within the nasal cavity. Most occur in the anterior portions of the nose, but when a posterior bleed occurs, it is likely to persist because it may be arterial in nature.

More than 90% of incidents are caused by local irritation related to trauma or inflammation. Local causes include injury and irritation, septal abnormality, inflammation, and lesions. It is also associated with systemic causes such as blood dyscrasias, arteriosclerosis, and hereditary hemorrhagic telangiectasia.

Where It Occurs

- Most common in children under age 10 and adults over age 50.
- Approximately 10% of the population experiences at least one significant nosebleed in a lifetime.
- Poorly humidified environments or high altitudes can increase likelihood of occurrence.

Signal Symptoms

- Blood in the nares, unilateral or bilateral.
- Taste of blood.

BE SAFE! Nasal packing may be done for severe cases, but it is important that the airway is not compromised so that the patient has adequate breathing.

Diagnostic Tests

Test	What It Shows	Patient Problems/ Nursing Care
Partial prothrombin time or thromboplastin time	Helps determine platelet-related coagulopathies and clotting factor disorders	Knowledge deficit: explain procedures. Patient will need venipuncture.
Complete blood count	Helps determine chronicity of the condition	Knowledge deficit: explain procedures. Patient will need venipuncture.

Treatment and Nursing Care

Potential Nursing Diagnoses*

Pain (acute)
Risk for infection
Knowledge deficit (medications, need for humidity)
Impaired skin integrity

BE SMART! If the patient is placed on antibiotics, make sure s/he takes the entire course of antibiotics.

■ After stopping the bleeding, treat the underlying cause as appropriate.
■ Treatment may include nasal packing, particularly for posterior bleeds. Note that posterior packing can lead to pain. Usually antibiotics are needed because the packing can lead to toxic shock syndrome in rare cases.
■ Avoid giving pain medications that will decrease platelet function and increase bleeding such as NSAIDs.
■ Other treatment: cauterization, arterial ligation, or embolization.

Retinal Detachment

A retinal detachment is an emergency that occurs when the retina is pulled away from or out of its normal position. The most common cause of retinal detachment is the formation of a hole or tear, which can occur as part of the normal aging process or during cataract surgery or trauma. The hole allows the vitreous fluid to leak out between the layers, separating the sensory retinal layer from its blood supply in the choroid.

Retinal detachments are classified as rhegmatogenous, tractional, and exudative. A rhegmatogenous retinal detachment, the most common form, is a retinal tear leading to fluid accumulation and separation of the neurosensory retina from the underlying retinal pigment epithelium. With a tractional detachment, contractile membranes pull the neurosensory retina away from the retinal pigment epithelium. Exudative detachment occurs with a change in the inflow or outflow of fluid from the vitreous cavity that leads to fluid accumulation in the subretinal space.

Where It Occurs

- A retinal detachment most often occurs in women and men between ages 50 and 70.
- Of those less than 45 years of age, the prevalence is higher in males than in females.
- Associated with congenital malformations, injury and trauma, previous eye surgery, tumors, disease of the vitreous humor, and degeneration of eye structures.

Signal Symptoms

- A painless change in vision with flashing lights, black spots ("floaters"); shower of black spots.
- Shadows in the peripheral visual field; visual distortion; cobwebs sensation.

BE SAFE! As vision changes in older adults, it increases the risk of falls and injury.

Diagnostic Tests

Test	What It Tells	Patient Problems/ Nursing Care
Ophthalmoscopic examination	Gray bulge or fold in retina is visible, indicating that the retina is detached	Knowledge deficit: explain all procedures.

Treatment and Nursing Care

Potential Nursing Diagnoses*

Disturbed sensory perception (visual)
Anxiety
Ineffective coping

BE SMART! Explain all treatment options to the patient.

- Cyclopentolate hydrochloride (Cyclogyl) to dilate the pupil and rest the muscles of accommodation.
- Antibiotics to prevent eye infections.
- Recommend a referral to a retinal-vitreous specialist.
- Surgical repair, in which the retina is forced into contact with the choroid to enable the scleral buckling procedure to place the retina back into position, is required for a detached retina.
- Laser therapy and cryotherapy (ambulatory outpatient procedures).
- Make sure patient understands all postoperative management including activity restrictions and signs of complications.

Stomatitis

Stomatitis is a recurrent, self-limiting condition characterized by painful ulcerative eruptions of the oral mucosa and tongue and is the most common oral lesion. It is also called *aphthous stomatitis, recurrent aphthous ulcers (RAUs)*, or *canker sores*. It may involve either a portion of or the entire oral cavity.

The cause of the condition is unknown but is believed to involve an aberrant immune response triggered by any number of environmental or immune-related factors, including viral infections, genetic predisposition, nutritional (hematinic) deficiency (iron, folic acid, vitamins B_6 and B_{12}), immune suppression, and bacterial infection.

Where It Occurs

- Occurs in adults of all ages, with peak initial onset between ages 10 and 19. As people age, the sores tend to diminish.
- Women are more commonly affected than men.
- People who wear dentures (*denture stomatitis*) and smoke (*nicotine stomatitis*) are at risk.
- People with systemic lupus erythematosus and inflammatory bowel disease are at risk.

Signal Symptoms

- Prodrome burning, pricking, or tightening sensation in the mouth prior to appearance of ulcers.
- Ulcers can be shallow or deep, more than 1 cm in diameter, and appear singly or in clusters.
- Pain in the mouth.

BE SAFE! Avoid foods that might injure the oral mucosa and sharp eating implements that might disrupt the tissues.

Diagnostic Tests

Diagnostic tests can be used to rule out differential diagnoses.

Test	What It Tells	Patient Problems/ Nursing Care
Vitamin B_{12}, folate, and iron levels	Determine presence of nutritional deficiencies	Knowledge deficit: explain procedures. Patient will need venipuncture.
Complete blood count and differential	Rules out anemias and neutropenia	Knowledge deficit: explain procedures. Patient will need venipuncture.

Treatment and Nursing Care

Potential Nursing Diagnoses*

Impaired mucous membrane integrity
Impaired tissue integrity
Risk for infection
Pain (acute)

BE SMART! Outbreaks may be related to stress and immune suppression. Teach patient techniques for stress reduction.

- Topical treatments may be used, but evidence for their efficacy is lacking: corticosteroids and immunomodulatory agents such as retinoids and cyclosporine may be used in gel, cream, or ointment form.
- Rinses such as hydrogen peroxide reduce bacteria; topical lidocaine or benzocaine may reduce pain.
- Teach patient to avoid salty and spicy foods, which may increase pain. Some patients state that pineapple, cinnamon, and nuts lead to additional outbreaks. Consider a nutritional consultation and multivitamins.

Acute Respiratory Distress Syndrome

Acute respiratory distress syndrome (ARDS), the most severe form of acute lung injury, is defined as noncardiogenic pulmonary edema that occurs despite low to normal pressures in the pulmonary capillaries. Various conditions can predispose a patient to ARDS, but they usually represent a sudden catastrophic situation. These conditions can be classified into two categories: direct lung injury and indirect lung injury. Direct injury occurs from situations such as gastric aspiration, near drowning, chemical inhalation, and oxygen toxicity. Indirect injury occurs from mediators released during sepsis, multiple trauma, thermal injury, hypoperfusion or hemorrhagic shock, disseminated intravascular coagulation, drug overdose, and massive blood transfusions.

As ARDS progresses, patients exhibit decreased lung volumes and markedly decreased lung compliance. Type II pneumocytes, the cells responsible for surfactant production, are damaged. This deficiency is thought to be partly responsible for the alveolar collapse and the decrease in lung volumes that occur. In addition, fibroblasts proliferate in the alveolar wall, migrate into the intra-alveolar fluid, and ultimately convert the exudate (fluid with high concentration of protein and cellular debris) into fibrous tissue. Refractory hypoxemia occurs as the lungs are perfused but not ventilated (a condition called capillary shunting) owing to the damage to the alveoli and developing fibrosis. Respiratory failure and cardiopulmonary arrest can develop.

Where It Occurs

■ ARDS can occur equally across genders and at any age, including during childhood, to those who have been subjected to severe physiological stresses such as sepsis, burns, or trauma.

Signal Symptoms

■ Acute respiratory distress, rapid respiratory rate, increase in the work of breathing, nasal flaring, the use of accessory muscles to breathe, and diaphoresis.
■ If ARDS has progressed: dusky appearance, cyanosis around the lips and nailbeds, pallor.

BE SAFE! ARDS progresses rapidly. Monitor that the patient has an open airway and adequate gas exchange.

Diagnostic Tests

The diagnosis of ARDS can be controversial and is one of exclusion.

Test	What It Tells	Patient Problems/ Nursing Care
Chest x-ray	Findings reflect noncardiogenic pulmonary edema	Knowledge deficit: explain procedures.
Arterial blood gases (ABGs)	Findings demonstrate poor gas exchange that leads to hypoxemia and, as respiratory failure progresses, to hypercapnia	Pain (acute); if the patient does not have arterial catheter, the arterial puncture is painful without topical anesthesia.

Treatment and Nursing Care

Potential Nursing Diagnoses*

Impaired gas exchange
Ineffective breathing pattern
Ineffective airway clearance
Risk for infection

BE SMART! Monitor the patient's oxygenation with a pulse oximeter.

- Intubation and mechanical ventilation.
- Sedation.
- To augment gas exchange, the patient needs endotracheal suctioning periodically.
- Turn the patient as often as possible, even every hour, to increase ventilation and perfusion to all areas of the lung.
- May be given nitric oxide to decrease pulmonary vascular resistance with increased perfusion to ventilated areas.

Asthma

Asthma is classified as an intermittent, reversible, obstructive disease of the lungs. It is characterized by airway inflammation and hyperreactivity (increased responsiveness to a wide variety of triggers). Hyperreactivity leads to airway obstruction due to acute onset of muscle spasm in the smooth muscle of the tracheobronchial tree, thereby leading to a narrowed lumen. In addition to muscle spasm, there is swelling of the mucosa, which leads to edema. Lastly, the mucous glands increase in number, hypertrophy, and secrete thick mucus.

The main triggers for asthma are allergies, viral infections, autonomic nervous system imbalances that can cause an increase in parasympathetic stimulation, medications, psychological factors, and exercise. Of asthmatic conditions in patients under 30 years old, 70% are caused by allergies. Three major indoor allergens are dust mites, cockroaches, and cats. In older patients, the cause is almost always nonallergic types of irritants such as smog. Heredity plays a part in about one-third of the cases.

Where It Occurs

- Although the incidence of asthma is estimated at 1% to 5% in the general population, children have a higher incidence of 12%.
- Asthma is diagnosed more frequently in males under 14 years and over 45 years of age and in females between ages 15 and 45.

Signal Symptoms

- Mild intermittent: less than twice a week (cough, wheeze, chest tightness, difficulty breathing) with brief flare-ups of varying intensity, no symptoms between flare-ups, and nighttime symptoms less than twice a month.
- Mild persistent: three to six times a week (cough, wheeze, chest tightness, difficulty breathing) with flare-ups that may affect activity level and nighttime symptoms three to four times a month.
- Moderate persistent: daily (cough, wheeze, chest tightness, difficulty breathing) with flare-ups that may affect activity level and nighttime symptoms five or more times a month.
- Severe persistent: continual (cough, wheeze, chest tightness, difficulty breathing) with frequent nighttime symptoms.

BE SAFE! Asthma kills. Make sure patient has a patent airway with gas exchange.

Diagnostic Tests

Test	What It Tells	Patient Problems/ Nursing Care
Forced vital capacity (FVC): maximum volume of air that can be forcefully expired after a maximal lung inspiration	Lower than normal result because airway obstruction decreases flow rates	Knowledge deficit: explain procedures. Results of this test are effort dependent.
Forced expiratory volume in 1 second (FEV_1): volume of air expired in 1 second from the beginning of the FVC maneuver	Lower than normal result because airway obstruction decreases flow rates	Knowledge deficit: explain procedures. Results of this test are effort dependent.

Treatment and Nursing Care

Potential Nursing Diagnoses*

Ineffective airway clearance
Impaired gas exchange
Ineffective breathing pattern
Knowledge deficit (medications, lifestyle, allergens, exercise)

BE SMART! Because patients (especially children) with asthma have a history of allergies, obtain a thorough description of the response to allergens or other irritants.

- Bronchodilators, such as albuterol, using a metered-dose inhaler (MDI) to reverse airflow obstruction.
- Systemic corticosteroids to decrease inflammatory response.
- Maintenance of airway, breathing, and circulation is the primary consideration during an acute attack.
- Patients often require intravenous fluid replacement.
- Teach avoidance of allergens.
- Teach asthma self management.

Cancer, Breast

Breast cancer, the most frequently diagnosed serious cancer and leading cause of cancer death among women, is classified as either noninvasive or invasive. Noninvasive carcinoma refers to cancer in the ducts or lobules and is also called carcinoma in situ (5% of breast cancers). Invasive carcinoma (also known as infiltrating carcinoma) occurs when the cancer cells invade the tissue beyond the ducts or lobules. Carcinoma of the breast stems from the epithelial tissues of the ducts and lobules. Ductal carcinoma is the most common type of breast cancer.

The origin of breast cancer is a complex interaction between the biologic and endocrine properties of the person and the environmental exposures that may precipitate mutation of cells to a malignancy. The greatest risk by far is family history of breast cancer. Survival rates for breast cancer have continued to increase, especially in younger women. Recent breast cancer research has led to progress with improved and less toxic management strategies.

Where It Occurs

■ Annual incidence of breast cancer is less than 60 per 100,000 below age 40; 100 per 100,000 by age 50; and nearly 200 per 100,000 at age 70.
■ Only 1% of breast cancer affects men, and it usually occurs when they are over age 60.

Signal Symptoms

■ Breast cancer may be without symptoms in the early stages.
■ Inflammation, dimpling, orange peel effect, distended vessels, and nipple changes or ulceration are all indications of advanced disease.

BE SAFE! Before a lump is felt, breast cancer is often detected not by symptoms but as an abnormal mammogram.

Diagnostic Tests

Test	What It Tells	Patient Problems/ Nursing Care
Mammogram	Shows a radio-dense or white mass, which suggests a diagnosis of cancer	Knowledge deficit: explain procedures.
Ultrasound of the breast	Reveals a white lesion that can differentiate between cystic and solid lesions	Knowledge deficit: explain procedures.

Treatment and Nursing Care

Potential Nursing Diagnoses*

Body image disturbance
Anxiety
Ineffective sexuality pattern
Knowledge deficit (medications, pre- and postoperative management)

BE SMART! Evaluation of breast cancer is considered a triple assessment: clinical examination, imaging (mammography or ultrasonography), and needle biopsy.

- Treatment is based on the stage of disease at diagnosis according to the TNM classification (T = tumor size, N = involvement of regional lymph nodes, M = metastasis).
- The goal of surgery is control of cancer in breast and axillary nodes.
- Most women have a choice of surgical procedures; depends on the clinical stage, tumor location, contraindications to radiation.
- Radiotherapy given 2 to 4 weeks after breast-preserving surgery for stages I and II breast cancer.
- Combination chemotherapy is recommended for pre- and postmenopausal patients with positive nodes. Hormonal therapy is used to change the levels of hormones that promote cancer growth and increase survival time in women with metastatic breast cancer.

Cancer, Laryngeal

The cause of laryngeal cancer is unknown, but the two major predisposing factors are prolonged use of alcohol and tobacco. Each substance poses an independent risk, but their combined use causes a synergistic effect. Other risk factors include a familial tendency, a history of frequent laryngitis or vocal straining, chronic inhalation of noxious fumes, poor nutrition, human papillomavirus, and a weakened immune system.

About 95% of all laryngeal cancers are squamous cell carcinomas; adenocarcinomas and sarcomas account for the other 5%. Most cases of laryngeal cancer are diagnosed before metastasis occurs. If it is confined to the glottis (the true vocal cords), laryngeal cancer usually grows slowly and metastasizes late because of the limited lymphatic drainage of the cords. Sixty percent of the cancers begin in the glottis, 35% begin in the supraglottis, and 5% begin in the subglottis. Laryngeal cancer that involves the supraglottis (false vocal cords) and subglottis (a rare downward extension from the vocal cords) tends to metastasize early to the lymph nodes in the neck because of the rich lymphatic drainage of this area.

Where It Occurs

- More common in men than in women (5:1 ratio).
- Occurs most frequently between ages 50 and 70.

Signal Symptoms

- Early: a change (hoarseness, shortness of breath, pain) in the quality of people's voices.
- Late: dysphagia, persistent cough, hemoptysis, weight loss, dyspnea, or pain that radiates to the ear.

BE SAFE! Maintaining a patent airway is the highest priority during diagnosis and management.

Diagnostic Tests

Test	What It Tells	Patient Problems/ Nursing Care
Nasopharyngoscopy/ laryngoscopy	Cancers of the oral cavity and nasopharynx are visible	Knowledge deficit: explain procedures. NPO prior to procedure, and patient may experience sore throat.
Panendoscopy	Cancers of the larynx, hypopharynx, esophagus, trachea, and bronchi are visible	Knowledge deficit: explain procedures. NPO prior to procedure.

Treatment and Nursing Care

Potential Nursing Diagnoses*

Ineffective airway clearance
Impaired verbal communication
Disturbed body image
Pain (acute and chronic)
Impaired swallowing

BE SMART! Provide analgesia to help the patient maintain pain-free status.

- Analgesics, such as morphine sulfate and fentanyl, to relieve pain.
- The two types of therapy commonly used are radiation therapy and surgery.
- After surgery, the patient should have an alternative means of communication at all times.
- Patient education needed for ongoing cancer surveillance, medications, and communication strategies.

Chest Tubes

Chest tubes (tube thoracostomy) are inserted into the pleural cavity after a patient has suffered a collapsed lung. Conditions that might lead to chest tube insertion include pneumothorax, empyema, hemothorax, and pleural effusion. Traumatic pneumothorax can also be classified as either open (when atmospheric air enters the pleural space) or closed (when air enters the pleural space from the lung).

Chest tubes re-establish normal lung mechanics. During inspiration, negative intrathoracic pressure draws air into the lungs and is maintained in the pleural space (potential space between the parietal and visceral layers of the lung's pleura). When air, fluid, or blood accumulates in the pleural space, the pressure in the plural space becomes positive and insufficient ventilation and even lung collapse can occur. Tube thoracostomy re-establishes negative pressure in the pleural space to allow for normal ventilation.

Where It Occurs

- Pneumothorax can occur at any age.
- Elderly people with COPD and younger people with paraseptal emphysema are susceptible to spontaneous pneumothorax.

Signal Symptoms

- Chest pain, shortness of breath, difficulty in breathing, fatigue.
- Patients with an open pneumothorax also exhibit a sucking sound on inspiration.

BE SAFE! Open traumatic pneumothorax constitutes a life-threatening emergency and needs to be managed immediately.

Diagnostic Tests

Test	What It Tells	Patient Problems/ Nursing Care
Chest x-ray	Displays collapsed lung	Knowledge deficit: explain procedures.

Treatment and Nursing Care

Potential Nursing Diagnoses*

Impaired gas exchange
Ineffective breathing pattern
Pain (acute)
Risk for infection

BE SMART! Chest tubes are painful. Provide analgesia.

- Chest tubes are placed in the triangle of safety (anterior border of latissimus dorsi, the lateral border of pectoralis major, and a horizontal line lateral at the level of the fifth intercostal space).
- Monitor tube unit for any kinks or bubbling, which could indicate an air leak.
- Place the patient in a semi-Fowler's position to improve lung expansion.
- Secure all connections of the chest tube system with tape.
- Ensure the correct position of the underwater seal bottle or the disposable system. If a bottle is used, it should be erect and at least 100 cm below the level of the patient's chest.

Chronic Obstructive Pulmonary Disease

Chronic obstructive pulmonary disease (COPD) includes a group of disorders characterized by airflow obstruction that affects 32 million people in the United States. It is the fourth leading cause of death. The two most common disorders are emphysema and chronic bronchitis, which can occur alone or in combination, as well as asthma.

The primary sites of changes in COPD are the large airways of the lungs as well as the small bronchioles and the lung functional tissue, the parenchyma. The most common cause of COPD is cigarette smoke, which leads to an amplified inflammatory response. The inflammatory response leads to release of large numbers of activated polymorphonuclear leukocytes and macrophages. These cells release enzymes such as elastases that destroy functional lung tissue, resulting in inflamed airways; increased mucous production; damaged endothelium; and, in emphysema, enlarged airspaces distal to the terminal bronchioles.

Where It Occurs

- Incidence increases with age.
- The onset of chronic bronchitis usually occurs after age 35.
- Symptoms of emphysema occur after age 50.
- In addition to smoking, causes include traffic pollution, occupational exposure to toxic inhaled substances, and genetic causes.

Signal Symptoms

- Chronic bronchitis: chronic cough productive of sputum (for at least 3 months for 2 consecutive years), shortness of breath, frequent pulmonary infections.
- Emphysema: dyspnea on exertion, diminished breath sounds, distant heart sounds.
- Asthma: breathlessness, wheezing.

BE SAFE! COPD is becoming more common in women due to the increased incidence of smoking in women.

Diagnostic Tests

Test	What It Tells	Patient Problems/ Nursing Care
Chest x-ray	Seldom diagnostic but may rule out other pathology	Knowledge deficit: explain procedures.
Pulmonary function tests	Show decreased lung capacity	Knowledge deficit: explain procedures. Recognize that results are effort dependent.

Treatment and Nursing Care

Potential Nursing Diagnoses*

Ineffective airway clearance
Ineffective breathing pattern
Activity intolerance
Risk for infection

- Overall goal: improve a patient's functional status and quality of life by preserving lung function.
- Bronchodilators: anticholinergic agents, beta-adrenergic agents, and theophylline.
- Management of inflammation with inhaled and systemic corticosteroids.
- Treatment includes avoidance of contributing factors, prevention or early recognition and treatment of respiratory infections, bronchodilation, aggressive management of acute exacerbations, and oxygen therapy.
- Teach patient about lifestyle management, including active pulmonary rehabilitation.

Hemothorax

Hemothorax, an accumulation of blood in the pleural space, affects oxygenation, ventilation, and hemodynamic stability. Most instances of hemothorax are caused by blunt trauma from motor vehicle crashes (MVCs), assaults, and falls or by penetrating trauma from knives or gunshot wounds. Oxygenation is affected because the accumulation of blood exerts pressure on pulmonary structures, leading to alveolar collapse, a decreased surface area for gas exchange, and impaired diffusion of oxygen from the alveolus to the blood. Ventilation is likewise impaired as the accumulating blood takes the place of gas in the lungs. Hemodynamic instability occurs as bleeding increases in the pleural space and vascular volume is depleted. Pneumothorax, or air in the pleural cavity, often accompanies hemothorax.

The hemorrhage can occur from pulmonary parenchymal lacerations, intercostal artery lacerations, or disruptions of the pulmonary or bronchial vasculature. Low pulmonary pressures and thromboplastin in the lungs may aid in spontaneously tamponading parenchymal lacerations. Complications of hemothorax include hypovolemic shock, exsanguination, organ failure, cardiopulmonary arrest, and death. Some experts define a hemothorax only when the hematocrit is greater than 50%, as compared to a bloody pleural effusion, but most do not differentiate between the two conditions.

Where It Occurs

■ Because trauma is the leading cause of death in the first four decades of life, hemothorax is most commonly seen in children and young adults.
■ Chest trauma occurs in about 60% of all multitrauma patients.

Signal Symptoms

■ Paradoxical chest movement; affected side of the chest may fall instead of rising with inspiration due to lack of support structure.
■ Absent breath sounds on side of injury; dullness to percussion due to accumulation of blood.
■ Bruising and lacerations over the chest wall; in drivers of car crashes, imprint of steering wheel may be visible.

BE SAFE! A collapsed lung is an emergency because of the risk of hypoxemia, or tension pneumothorax, which causes collapse of the unaffected lung due to buildup of pressure in the thoracic cavity.

Diagnostic Tests

Test	What It Tells	Patient Problems/ Nursing Care
Chest x-ray	Opacity at the area of bleeding and lung collapse determines location and extent	Knowledge deficit: explain procedures.
Complete blood count	Decreased values reflective of the degree of hemorrhage	Knowledge deficit: explain procedures. Patient will need venipuncture.

Potential Nursing Diagnoses*

Ineffective breathing pattern
Ineffective airway clearance
Pain (acute)
Fluid volume deficit
Anxiety
Risk for infection

BE SMART! Clots may occlude the chest tube draining system, leading to a buildup of fluid and recollapse of the lung. Keep the chest tube patent and free flowing without kinks.

- Treatment of a hemothorax focuses on stabilizing the patient's condition by maintaining airway and breathing, stopping the bleeding, emptying blood from the pleural cavity, and re-expanding the underlying lung by tube thoracostomy.
- Antibiotics to protect from or combat bacterial infections.
- Analgesics to reduce pain and increase mobility.
- Nursing care includes ensuring that chest tube is patent and draining freely. The processes of "milking" or "stripping" chest tubes are controversial, but most evidence shows that the procedures do not improve outcomes and may cause discomfort and injury to the patient.

Influenza

Influenza (flu) is an acute, highly contagious viral respiratory infection caused by one of three types of myxovirus influenzae. Influenzavirus A causes the most serious epidemics. Influenzavirus B produces milder respiratory infections. Influenzavirus C causes mild respiratory infections like the common cold.

Influenza is usually a self-limited disease that lasts from 2 to 7 days. Complications include pneumonia, myositis, exacerbation of chronic obstructive pulmonary disease, and Reye's syndrome. In rare cases, influenza can lead to encephalitis, transverse myelitis, myocarditis, pericarditis, or even death.

Where It Occurs

- The incidence of influenza cases is highest in school-age children and generally decreases with age. During an outbreak of the disease, however, elderly persons and those disabled by chronic illnesses are most likely to develop severe complications.
- Males and females of all races/ethnicities and all ages are affected.

Signal Symptoms

- The patient's temperature usually ranges from 102°F to 103°F and often rises suddenly on the first day before falling and rising again on the third day of illness. Headache, weakness, fatigue, cough, rhinitis, nausea, vomiting, diarrhea.
- Increased respirations, fatigue, myalgias; redness of the soft palate, tonsils, and pharynx.

BE SAFE! If the patient does not improve after 5 to 7 days or has prolonged fever, complications may be occurring, and the patient may need to see a health-care provider for a change in therapy.

Diagnostic Tests

No specific diagnostic tests are used because diagnosis is made by the history of symptoms and onset. If the patient has symptoms of a bacterial infection that complicates influenza, cultures and sensitivities may be required.

Treatment and Nursing Care

Potential Nursing Diagnoses*

Risk for infection
Fluid volume deficit
Pain (acute)
Activity intolerance
Hyperthermia

BE SMART! Influenza vaccine provides good protection against many strains and is effective approximately 2 weeks after administration.

- Bedrest and increased intake of fluids are prescribed for patients in the acute stage of infection.
- Antipyretics control fever and discomfort; however, aspirin is generally avoided to reduce the risk of Reye's syndrome.
- Amantadine provides antiviral action against influenza (prophylaxis and symptomatic); usually prescribed for outbreaks of influenza A within a closed population, such as a nursing home.
- The most important nursing intervention is prevention.

Pleural Effusion

The pleural space generally contains only 1 ml of fluid; a pleural effusion is the collection of an unusually large amount of fluid there. Symptoms result from fluid in the pleural space, which occurs as a consequence of limited fluid absorption or increased production. It is the most common effect of pleural disease. Pleural effusions can be the result of either a pulmonary or nonpulmonary disease. Causes include heart failure, cirrhosis, atelectasis, nephritic syndrome, constrictive pericarditis, and myxedema.

Where It Occurs

- Because pleural effusions develop as part of an underlying disease, they typically are found in individuals more likely to contract the causative disorder. Pleural effusions are typically found in adults.

Signal Symptoms

- With smaller effusions, no physical findings are generally evident. With larger effusions, symptoms include dyspnea, cough, and chest pain; findings include dullness to percussion, pleural friction rub, and decreased breath.
- Hypoxemia (restlessness, confusion, tachycardia, cyanosis), bloody sputum, chest wall pain, pleuritic chest pain.

BE SAFE! A pleural effusion, if large enough, can compress the lungs and reduce gas exchange.

Diagnostic Tests

Test	What It Tells	Patient Problems/ Nursing Care
Chest x-ray	Shows normal or abnormal chest structures	Knowledge deficit: explain all procedures.
Analysis of pleuritic fluid	Shows the presence of bacteria, pus, fat, or blood	Knowledge deficit: explain all procedures. Manage pain and support patient during procedure.

Treatment and Nursing Care

Potential Nursing Diagnoses*

Ineffective breathing patterns
Pain (acute)
Impaired physical mobility
Anxiety
Risk for infection

BE SMART! If patient needs a chest tube for drainage, monitor the amount and nature of the drainage.

- Pleural effusions are often treated by addressing the underlying disorder.
- Needle thoracentesis, video-assisted thoracoscopy with visualization and biopsy of the pleura. Other surgical procedures include surgical shunts and decortication.
- If infection is present, patient will need antibiotics. Make sure patient understands all medications and treatment options.
- Monitor the chest tube drainage system for air leaks.

Pneumonia

Pneumonia is an inflammatory condition of the interstitial lung tissue in which fluid and blood cells escape into the alveoli. The disease process begins with an infection in the alveolar spaces. As the organism multiplies, the alveolar spaces fill with fluid, white blood cells, and cellular debris from phagocytosis of the infectious agent. The infection spreads from the alveolus and can involve the distal airways (bronchopneumonia), part of a lobe (lobular pneumonia), or an entire lung (lobar pneumonia).

The inflammatory process causes the lung tissue to stiffen, resulting in a decrease in lung compliance and an increase in the work of breathing. The fluid-filled alveoli cause a physiological shunt, and venous blood passes unventilated portions of lung tissue and returns to the left atrium unoxygenated. As the arterial oxygen tension falls, the patient begins to exhibit the signs and symptoms of hypoxemia. In addition to hypoxemia, pneumonia can lead to respiratory failure and septic shock. Infection may spread via the bloodstream and cause endocarditis, pericarditis, meningitis, or bacteremia.

Primary pneumonia is caused by the patient's inhaling or aspirating a pathogen such as bacteria or a virus. Bacterial pneumonia, often caused by staphylococcus, streptococcus, or *Klebsiella*, usually occurs when the lungs' defense mechanisms are impaired by such factors as suppressed cough reflex, decreased cilia action, decreased activity of phagocytic cells, and the accumulation of secretions. Secondary pneumonia ensues from lung damage that was caused by the spread of bacteria from an infection elsewhere in the body or by a noxious chemical. Aspiration pneumonia is caused by the patient's inhaling foreign matter such as food or vomitus into the bronchi.

Where It Occurs

- People over 40 years of age are at greater risk to contract all forms of bacterial pneumonia, with older men more susceptible to streptococcal bacterial pneumonia and *Klebsiella* bacterial pneumonia.
- Older people are also at greater risk for viral pneumonia caused by influenza.
- Neonates with multisystem disease are also at risk for viral pneumonia caused by cytomegalovirus.

Signal Symptoms

- Fever, tachypnea, dyspnea, accessory muscle use during breathing, tachycardia, central cyanosis.
- Altered mental status, irritability, restlessness.
- Rales, crackles, rhonchi, or wheezes; decreased breath sounds.

- Areas in the chest of consolidation or tactile fremitus.
- Changes in breathing, such as rales, crackles, rhonchi, and wheezes; E to A changes; and whispered pectoriloquy.

> **BE SAFE!** Make sure that the patient has an open airway and adequate breathing.

Diagnostic Tests

Test	What It Tells	Patient Problems/ Nursing Care
Rapid detection test: reverse-transcriptase-polymerase chain reaction	If positive, virus is present	Knowledge deficit: explain procedures.
Sputum cultures and sensitivities	Identifies and indicates presence of infecting organism and how resistant the bacteria are to antibiotics	Knowledge deficit: explain procedures.

Treatment and Nursing Care

Potential Nursing Diagnoses*

Ineffective airway clearance
Ineffective breathing pattern
Risk for activity tolerance
Fluid volume deficit
Pain (acute)

> **BE SMART!** For bacterial pneumonia, make sure the patient gets adequate rest, fluids, and antibiotics.

- A variety of antibiotics are prescribed for bacterial pneumonia and antivirals for viral pneumonia.
- Humidified oxygen; patient may need endotracheal intubation and mechanical ventilation. Corticosteroids may be used in emergency cases.
- Encourage coughing and deep breathing every 2 hours.

- Three liters of fluid should be consumed per day. Manage fever.
- Conserve the patient's energy by providing adequate rest during the acute phase.
- Teach the patient prevention strategies, how to achieve rest and rehabilitation, how to manage fever, and to take all medications.

Pneumothorax

Pneumothorax occurs when air accumulates in the pleural space. Pneumothorax increases intrapleural pressure, resulting in the collapse of the lung on the affected side. The three major types of pneumothorax are spontaneous, traumatic, and tension. Spontaneous pneumothorax is not life threatening. Traumatic pneumothorax can also be classified as either open (when atmospheric air enters the pleural space) or closed (when air enters the pleural space from the lung). Open traumatic pneumothorax constitutes a life-threatening emergency.

Tension pneumothorax is defined as the buildup of air within the pleural space, usually a potential space without air. Air is trapped in the pleural space without escape. Buildup of pressure pushes the mediastinum to the opposite side of the body, blocks venous return to the heart, and may cause cardiac and respiratory arrest.

The cause of a closed or primary spontaneous pneumothorax is the rupture of a bleb (vesicle) on the surface of the visceral pleura. Secondary spontaneous pneumothorax can result from chronic obstructive pulmonary disease (COPD), which is related to hyperinflation or air trapping, or from the effects of cancer, which can result in the weakening of lung tissue or erosion into the pleural space by the tumor. Blunt chest trauma and penetrating chest trauma are the primary causes of traumatic and tension pneumothorax. Other possible causes include therapeutic procedures such as thoracotomy, thoracentesis, and insertion of a central line.

Where It Occurs

- Elderly people with COPD and younger people with paraseptal emphysema are susceptible to spontaneous pneumothorax.
- Spontaneous primary pneumothorax occurs most often in tall, thin men between ages 30 and 40.

- More men than women experience pneumothorax.
- Cigarette smoking predisposes people to pneumothorax.

Signal Symptoms

- Spontaneous pneumothorax usually occurs at rest; severe, stabbing chest pain and shortness of rest, anxiety, cough, fatigue.
- Open pneumothorax: sucking sound on inspiration, visible wound caused by a penetrating object, tachycardia, dyspnea, cardiovascular collapse.
- Tension pneumothorax: respiratory distress, dyspnea, cyanosis, apnea, hypotension, tachycardia, cardiac arrest; if intubated, difficulty in ventilation; mediastinal shift and tracheal deviation (classic sign not always seen clinically).

BE SAFE! Even small penetrating wounds can be life threatening if vital structures are perforated.

Diagnostic Tests

Test	What It Tells	Patient Problems/ Nursing Care
Chest x-ray	Confirms diagnosis by demonstrating that lungs are collapsed and not filled with air	Knowledge deficit: explain procedures.

Treatment and Nursing Care

Potential Nursing Diagnoses*

Impaired gas exchange
Ineffective breathing pattern
Pain (acute)
Risk for infection

BE SMART! Monitor carefully for a tension pneumothorax (absent breath sounds, tracheal deviation) if an occlusive dressing is used; it prevents air from escaping the lungs from around the chest tube insertion site.

- The priority is to maintain airway, breathing, and circulation; initiate CPR if needed.
- The most important interventions focus on re-inflating the lung by evacuating the pleural air.
- For patients with jeopardized gas exchange, chest tube insertion may be necessary to achieve lung re-expansion.
- Chest tubes are placed in the triangle of safety (anterior border of latissimus dorsi, the lateral border of pectoralis major, and a horizontal line lateral at the level of the fifth intercostal space).
- Monitor tube unit for any kinks or bubbling, which could indicate an air leak.
- Place the patient in a semi-Fowler's position to improve lung expansion.
- Encourage coughing and deep breathing to remove secretions.

Pulmonary Fibrosis

Pulmonary fibrosis is a restrictive lung disease in which alveolar inflation is reduced, thus impairing lung function. The alveoli are affected by fibrotic tissue, which may develop after inflammation, infection, or tissue damage. The resulting scarring and distortion of pulmonary tissue lead to serious compromise in gas exchange. Fibrosis leads to decreased lung compliance and increased elastic recoil, which increases the overall work of breathing and inefficient exchange of gases.

Idiopathic pulmonary fibrosis (IPF) is of unknown etiology and is characterized by a poor prognosis and no effective treatment. Pulmonary fibrosis can also occur from exposure to radiation or inhalation of noxious materials such as silica, asbestos, and coal dust. Other conditions, both pulmonary and nonpulmonary, can also lead to pulmonary fibrosis.

Where It Occurs

- Elderly patients or those exposed to risk factors for a prolonged period of time are at the greatest risk.
- The average age of patients who are diagnosed with pulmonary fibrosis is 50.

Signal Symptoms

- Nonspecific symptoms such as exertional dyspnea, fatigue, and nonproductive cough.
- Late: shallow, rapid breathing patterns; diminished or absent breath sounds or coarse crackles.
- Weight loss, low-grade fevers, joint pain, myalgias.

BE SAFE! Because pulmonary fibrosis in its late stages can cause cor pulmonale, check for signs of cardiac failure, such as distended neck veins, liver distention, and swelling of the lower extremities.

Diagnostic Tests

Test	What It Tells	Patient Problems/ Nursing Care
Chest x-ray	Demonstrates changed appearance of fibrotic areas by identifying interstitial infiltrates or ground glass pattern	Knowledge deficit: explain procedures.
High resolution computed tomography	Demonstrates changed appearance of fibrotic areas by illustrating reticular opacities, traction bronchiectasis, honeycombing, and alveolar distortion	Knowledge deficit: explain procedures.

Treatment and Nursing Care

Potential Nursing Diagnoses*

Ineffective breathing pattern
Activity intolerance
Fatigue
Pain (chronic)

BE SMART! Teach the patient about activity limits, conserving energy, and pain control for myalgias.

- To relieve breathing difficulties and correct hypoxia, most physicians prescribe low-flow oxygen therapy (2–4 L/min).
- Prednisone may decrease the inflammatory process.
- Cyclophosphamide (Cytoxan) reduces the white blood cell count, which causes a distinct drop in the total blood lymphocyte count.
- Focus on relieving respiratory difficulties and caring for the patient's emotional condition.

Pulmonary Hypertension

Pulmonary hypertension is diagnosed when the systolic pressure in the pulmonary artery exceeds 30 mm Hg. It is most commonly seen in pre-existing pulmonary or cardiac disease but may occur (although rarely) as a primary condition when it is produced by fibrosis and thickening of the vessel intima. An increase in resistance of the vessels in the pulmonary vasculature bed occurs secondary to hypoxemia (oxygen deficiency). Chronic hypoxemia produces hypertrophy of the medial muscle layer in the smaller branches of the pulmonary artery, which decreases the size of the vessel lumen. Vasoconstriction, the pulmonary system's response to hypoxemia, results in a pressure buildup in the right side of the heart because flow through the pulmonary system is impaired. When hypertension in the pulmonary system (measured as pulmonary vascular resistance) is greater than the ability of the right side of the heart to pump, the cardiac output falls and may cause shock.

The cause of primary pulmonary hypertension is unknown, but the disease tends to occur in families. Secondary pulmonary hypertension is caused by conditions that produce hypoxemia, such as chronic obstructive pulmonary disease, obesity, alveolar hypoventilation, smoke inhalation, and high altitude.

Where It Occurs

- Pulmonary hypertension is most commonly seen in the elderly person with cardiac or pulmonary disease.
- Idiopathic primary pulmonary hypertension tends to occur more often in women between 20 and 40 years of age.

Signal Symptoms

- Signs of right ventricular failure: jugular venous distention, increased central venous pressure, and peripheral edema.
- Hyperventilation, coughing, rapid breathing (tachypnea) or dyspnea.
- Weakness, fatigue, sleep disturbance, syncope.

BE SAFE! Protect patient from falls during syncopal attacks.

Diagnostic Tests

Test	What It Tells	Patient Problems/ Nursing Care
Echocardiogram	Estimates ventricular functioning; pulmonary hypertension may occur because of right-to-left shunting across a patent foramen ovale	Knowledge deficit: explain procedures.
Pulmonary artery pressure and pulmonary vascular resistance (PVR)— measurements made with a pulmonary artery catheter	Demonstrates sustained elevation of pulmonary vascular pressures	Knowledge deficit: explain procedures. Check insertion site for bleeding and infection.

Treatment and Nursing Care

Potential Nursing Diagnoses*

Impaired gas exchange
Ineffective breathing pattern
Fatigue
Anxiety

BE SMART! Discuss treatment options with patient and family.

- If the origin of the problem is structural, surgery may be attempted. Heart-lung transplantation is a consideration for severe conditions.
- Diuretics reduce both right and left ventricular failure.
- Sodium warfarin (Coumadin) prevents microvascular thrombosis, venous stasis, and limitation of physical activity.
- Provide comfort measures in addition to any ordered medication.
- Patient may need support during diagnostic procedures. Make sure patient understands all medications and restrictions on lifestyle.

Restrictive Lung Disease

People with restrictive lung diseases have reduced lung volume because of changes in lung cells or in the lung pleura or chest wall. Characteristics include reduced total lung capacity (TLC) and vital capacity (VC) with normal airflow and normal airway resistance (functional residual capacity [FRC]).

Intrinsic (within the lung tissue) causes include inflammation or scarring of lung tissue (interstitial lung disease) or pneumonitis, idiopathic fibrotic diseases, connective-tissue diseases, drug-induced lung disease, and sarcoidosis. Extrinsic (outside the lung tissue) causes include nonmuscular diseases of the chest wall, kyphoscoliosis, and neuromuscular disorders.

Where It Occurs

- Generally the condition occurs in adults, with more women than men affected.
- More smokers than nonsmokers have restrictive lung disease.
- Sarcoidosis is related to genetics.

Signal Symptoms

- Intrinsic: exertional dyspnea, dry cough, hemoptysis, wheezing, pleuritic chest pain.
- Extrinsic: dyspnea, decreased exercise tolerance, frequent respiratory infections, muscle weakness, sleep-disordered breathing.
- Fatigue, dyspnea, increased secretions.

BE SAFE! Make sure patient has an open airway and adequate breathing.

Diagnostic Tests

Test	What It Tells	Patient Problems/ Nursing Care
Chest x-ray	Changes in lung pleura or chest wall	Knowledge deficit: explain procedures.

Treatment and Nursing Care

Potential Nursing Diagnoses*

Ineffective breathing pattern
Activity intolerance
Impaired physical mobility
Fatigue

BE SMART! Teach patient to schedule frequent rest periods to conserve energy and reduce fatigue until medications take effect.

- Medication management usually includes corticosteroids, immunosuppressive agents, and cytotoxic agents.
- Lung transplantation is considered for people who have refractory disease.
- Acute exacerbation occurs often; the primary presenting symptom is worsening dyspnea.
- Encourage patient to go to a smoking cessation class.
- Teach patient stress reduction techniques, how to conserve energy, and the dose and side effects of all medications.

Thoracic Aortic Aneurysm

A thoracic aortic aneurysm is an abnormal widening of the aorta between the aortic valve and the diaphragm. An aneurysm is defined as dilation of the aorta that is more than 150% of its normal diameter for a given segment. A diameter of greater than 3.5 cm is generally considered dilated for the thoracic aorta, whereas greater than 4.5 cm is considered aneurysmal.

Aneurysm formation is caused by a weakening of the medial layer of the aorta, which stretches outward, causing an outpouching of the aortic wall. Thoracic aortic aneurysms take four forms: fusiform, saccular, dissecting, and false aneurysms. The single most important cause is atherosclerosis.

Where It Occurs

- The most common thoracic aortic aneurysm is an ascending aortic aneurysm, which is usually seen in hypertensive men under 60 years of age.
- A descending aortic aneurysm is most common in elderly hypertensive men or younger patients with a history of traumatic chest injury.
- The incidence of thoracic aortic aneurysm is higher in men than in women by a ratio of 3:1 and is more common in whites than in other populations.

Signal Symptoms

- Ascending thoracic aortic aneurysm: most patients are not symptomatic until the aneurysm ruptures.
- Rupture: abdominal pain, hypotension, and a pulsatile abdominal mass.
- Contralateral (opposite side) difference in blood pressure; pericardial friction rub and aortic valve insufficiency murmur may be present, indicating the extension of an ascending aortic aneurysm proximally into the aortic valve.
- Descending: lower extremity ischemia, GI obstruction or bleeding, obstruction of the kidney ureters.

BE SAFE! A thoracic dissecting aneurysm may rupture into the pericardium, resulting in cardiac tamponade, hemorrhagic shock, and cardiac arrest.

Diagnostic Tests

Test	What It Tells	Patient Problems/ Nursing Care
Computed tomography scan	Locates outpouching within the aortic wall to assess size and location of aneurysm	Knowledge deficit: explain procedures.
Chest x-ray	May show widened mediastinum or enlarged calcified aortic shadow; a traumatic aneurysm may be associated with skeletal fractures	Knowledge deficit: explain procedures.

Treatment and Nursing Care

Potential Nursing Diagnoses*

Ineffective tissue perfusion (cerebral, cardiopulmonary, peripheral)
Decreased cardiac output
Ineffective airway clearance
Ineffective breathing pattern
Deficient fluid volume

BE SMART! Emergency care is essential with a ruptured aneurysm. Cardiopulmonary resuscitation may be necessary.

- A thoracic aortic aneurysm that is 4 cm in size or less may be treated with oral antihypertensives or a beta-blocking agent to control hypertension.
- A thoracic aortic aneurysm that is 5 cm or greater in diameter is usually treated surgically.
- Antihypertensives reduce blood pressure so that hypertension does not stress graft suture lines.
- Nitroprusside reduces blood pressure in acute or critical situations.
- Focus on maintaining adequate circulation, preventing complications, and implementing patient education.

Tuberculosis

Tuberculosis (TB) is an infectious disease caused by *Mycobacterium* tuberculosis, an aerobic acid-fast bacillus. Although it is most frequently a pulmonary disease, more than 15% of patients experience extrapulmonary TB that can infect the meninges, kidneys, bones, or other tissues. Pulmonary TB can range from a small infection of bronchopneumonia to diffuse, intense inflammation, necrosis, pleural effusion, and extensive fibrosis.

TB is transmitted by respiratory droplets through sneezing or coughing by an infected person. Most infected persons have had a sustained exposure to the active agent rather than a single one.

Where It Occurs

- TB is most common in the elderly population, in men than in women, and in those who are immunosuppressed (on corticosteroids or have HIV infection, cancer, malnutrition).
- In the United States, approximately 70% of TB cases occur among minorities.
- Other high-risk groups are hospital employees, urban dwellers, drug and alcohol abusers, nursing home residents, and people who are incarcerated.

Signal Symptoms

- Acutely ill appearance, fever, night sweats, muscle wasting, poor muscle tone, loss of subcutaneous fat, poor skin turgor, and dry flaky skin.
- Rapid heart rate, rapid and difficult breathing, and stridor.
- Diminished or absent breath sounds bilaterally or unilaterally from pleural effusion or pneumothorax, tubular breath sounds or whispered pectoriloquies over large lesions, crackles over the apex of the lungs during quick inspiration after a short cough.

BE SAFE! Use good hand-washing techniques and isolation to prevent the spread of TB.

Diagnostic Tests

Test	What It Tells	Patient Problems/ Nursing Care
Fluorochrome or acid-fast bacilli sputum	Positive result stemming from the fact that *Mycobacterium* tuberculosis resists decolorizing chemicals after staining	Knowledge deficit: explain procedures.
Chest x-ray	Radiographic assessment of the lungs to identify active TB or old lesions	Knowledge deficit: explain procedures.

Treatment and Nursing Care

Potential Nursing Diagnoses*

Risk of infection
Activity intolerance
Ineffective breathing pattern
Fatigue

BE SMART! Immunosuppressed patients or those undergoing immunosuppression therapy need to be tested for TB.

- Because TB typically becomes resistant to any single-drug therapy, patients generally receive a combination of drugs.
- Isoniazid inhibits synthesis of bacterial cell wall and hinders cell division.
- Rifampin interferes with RNA synthesis and can kill slower-growing organisms that reside in granuloma in lungs or other organs.
- Nursing priorities are to maintain and achieve adequate ventilation and oxygenation; prevent the spread of infection; support behaviors to maintain health; promote effective coping strategies; and provide information about the disease process, prognosis, and treatment needs.

Ventilatory Assist

Ventilators are classified by the way they cycle across their inspiratory and expiratory phases and are thereby considered volume-cycled, pressure-cycled, or time-cycled ventilators. Volume-cycled ventilators provide a consistent tidal volume with each breath. Pressure-cycled ventilators provide a preset pressure limit for every breath, and time-cycled ventilators provide tidal volume during a preset time. Indications for mechanical ventilation include slow or absent respirations, rapid ineffective respirations, respiratory fatigue, acute respiratory distress syndrome (ARDS), low vital capacity, hypoxemia, hypotension, unresponsiveness, and coma. Volume-cycled ventilators are the most commonly used with the assist-control mode. The assist-control mode has a tidal volume and rate preset and guaranteed, and yet the patient can determine, within limits, the frequency and timing of the breaths.

Ventilators have the following settings in addition to the type of ventilator: respiratory rate, fraction of inspired oxygen, inspiratory time, expiratory time, tidal volume (12 ml/kg body weight), and positive inspiratory pressure. Sometimes sighs are set, which are breaths 1.5 to 2 times the set tidal volume given 4 to 8 times an hour. Positive end-expiratory pressure may be used for alveolar collapse. Complications include barotrauma rupture of alveoli due to positive pressure ventilation), ventilator-associated pneumonia, and oxygen toxicity (damage to the alveoli from high levels of oxygen).

Where It Occurs

■ Mechanical ventilation is needed more often in older adults with acute and chronic diseases than in younger people.
■ Mechanical ventilation can occur both in the hospital and in the home with appropriate preparation.

Signal Symptoms

■ Dyspnea, apnea, shallow respirations, ineffective respirations, hypoxemia, hypercapnia.
■ Lack of a respiratory drive: drug overdose, coma, stroke.

BE SAFE! Maintain an open airway so that mechanical ventilation can occur.

Diagnostic Tests

Test	What It Tells	Patient Problems/ Nursing Care
Partial pressure of oxygen in arterial blood (PaO$_2$)	Hypoxemia occurs because of problems with ventilation and perfusion due to obstruction of pulmonary circulation	Knowledge deficit: explain procedures. Patient will need arterial puncture: warn patient that procedure is painful.

Treatment and Nursing Care

Potential Nursing Diagnoses*

Ineffective airway clearance
Ineffective breathing pattern
Impaired gas exchange
Anxiety
Knowledge deficit

BE SMART! Teach patient and family the rationale for mechanical ventilation and that the patient will not be able to speak while intubated.

- A pulmonologist will generally prescribe the ventilator settings in collaboration with nurses and respiratory therapists.
- Monitor arterial blood gases and/or pulse oximetry to ensure adequate gas exchange.
- As the patient's condition changes, ventilator settings must change.
- Patients generally need sedation to manage prolonged periods of intubation and mechanical ventilation.
- Weaning from the mechanical ventilator must be done slowly with careful monitoring.

Abdominal Aortic Aneurysm (AAA)

An abdominal aortic aneurysm (AAA) is a localized outpouching or dilation of the arterial wall in the latter portion of the descending segment of the aorta (infrarenal aorta). Aneurysms of the abdominal aorta occur more frequently than those of the thoracic aorta. AAA may be fusiform (spindle-shaped) or saccular (pouchlike) in shape. A fusiform aneurysm in which the dilated area encircles the entire aorta is most common. A saccular aneurysm has a dilated area on only one side of the vessel.

The outpouching of the wall of the aorta occurs when the musculoelastic middle layer or media of the artery becomes weak (often caused by plaque and cholesterol deposits) and degenerative changes occur. The inner and outer layers of the arterial wall are stretched, and as the pulsatile force of the blood rushes through the aorta, the vessel wall becomes increasingly weak, and the aneurysm enlarges. Abdominal aneurysms can be fatal. More than half of people with untreated aneurysms die of aneurysm rupture within 2 years.

Where It Occurs

- Abdominal aneurysms are far more common in hypertensive men than women; from three to eight times as many men as women develop AAA.
- They are 3.5 times more common in whites than in blacks/African Americans.
- The incidence of AAA increases with age. The occurrence is rare before age 50 and common between ages 60 and 80, when the atherosclerotic process tends to become more pronounced.

Signal Symptoms

- A pulsating abdominal mass in the periumbilical area, slightly to the left of midline with an audible bruit.
- Flank or back pain described as deep and steady.
- Epigastric discomfort, altered bowel patterns.

BE SAFE! Watch for signs that may indicate impending aneurysm rupture (shock, drop in blood pressure, tachycardia, cool skin, diaphoresis).

Diagnostic Tests

Test	What It Tells	Patient Problems/ Nursing Care
Standard test: abdominal ultrasonography for initial diagnosis	Tests for a widened aorta (>3 cm in diameter)	Knowledge deficit: explain procedure.
Computed tomography (CT) scan	Locates outpouching within the aortic wall and illustrates widened aorta >3 cm	Knowledge deficit: explain procedure.

Treatment and Nursing Care

Potential Nursing Diagnoses*

Fluid volume deficit (isotonic)
Ineffective tissue perfusion (peripheral)
Risk for infection
Knowledge deficit (postoperative monitoring)

> **BE SMART!** Make sure the patient has peripheral circulation to the legs and feet by checking peripheral pulses, noting skin temperature, and monitoring capillary refill.

- The treatment of choice for AAA 6 cm or greater in size is surgical repair.
- When aneurysms are smaller, they may be evaluated over time with ultrasound examination or CT scan, whereas other experts suggest elective surgical repair regardless of aneurysm size.
- Morphine and fentanyl may be used to relieve surgical pain.
- Postoperation, keep the incision clean and dry.

Angina

Angina is a symptom of ischemic heart disease characterized by paroxysmal and usually recurring substernal or precordial chest pain or discomfort. Angina is caused by varying combinations of increased myocardial demand

and decreased myocardial perfusion. The imbalance between supply and demand is caused either by a primary decrease in coronary blood flow or by a disproportionate increase in myocardial oxygen requirements. Blood flow through the coronary arteries is partially or completely obstructed because of coronary artery spasm, fixed stenosing plaques, disrupted plaques, thrombosis, platelet aggregation, and embolization.

Angina can be classified as chronic exertional (stable, typical) angina, variant angina (Prinzmetal's), unstable or crescendo angina, or silent ischemia. Chronic exertional angina is usually caused by obstructive coronary artery disease that causes the heart to be vulnerable to further ischemia under increased demand or workload. Variant angina may occur in people with normal coronary arteries who have cyclically recurring angina at rest, unrelated to effort. Unstable angina is diagnosed in patients who report a changing character, duration, and intensity of their pain. Experts are also recognizing that not all ischemic events are perceived by patients even though such events, called silent ischemia, may have adverse implications for the patient.

Where It Occurs

- The risk of ischemic heart disease increases with age and when predispositions to atherosclerosis (smoking, hypertension, diabetes mellitus, hyperlipoproteinemia) are present.
- In Americans 40 to 74 years old, the age-adjusted prevalence of angina is higher among women than men. In addition, atypical presentations of angina are also more common among women than men.
- In women older than 20 years, angina occurs in 3.9% of non-Hispanic white women, 6.2% of non-Hispanic black women, and 5.5% of Hispanic/Latina American women.

Signal Symptoms

- Chest discomfort is often described as an ache rather than an actual pain and may be characterized as a heaviness, pressure, tightness, squeezing sensation, or indigestion. The discomfort is typically located in the substernal region or across the anterior upper chest.
- Anginal discomfort of short duration, usually 3 to 5 minutes, but can last up to 30 minutes or longer.

BE SAFE! Manage chest pain immediately with medications and rest to decrease oxygen consumption.

Diagnostic Tests

Test	What It Tells	Patient Problems/ Nursing Care
Electrocardiogram (ECG)	Assesses the electrical conduction system, which is adversely affected by myocardial ischemia	Knowledge deficit: explain procedure and ask patient to rest quietly during procedure.
Creatine kinase isoenzyme (MB-CK)	One-third of patients with unstable angina may have elevations due to tissue damage	Knowledge deficit: explain procedures. Patient will need venipuncture.

Treatment and Nursing Care

Potential Nursing Diagnoses*

Ineffective tissue perfusion (cardiopulmonary)
Pain (acute)
Anxiety
Knowledge deficit (medications, diet, exercise)

BE SMART! Document the location, duration, type, and nature of the pain and the results of your interventions.

- For any patient who is experiencing an acute anginal episode, pain management is the priority not only for patient comfort but also to decrease myocardial oxygen consumption.
- Nitroglycerin relieves ischemic symptoms by vasodilation of coronary arteries and reduces left ventricular preload and afterload.
- Aspirin inhibits platelet aggregation to reduce risk of coronary artery blockage.
- To decrease oxygen demand, encourage the patient to maintain bedrest until the pain subsides.
- Initiate teaching about medications, activity and exercise, diet, stress reduction, smoking cessation, alcohol moderation.

Arterial Occlusive Disease

Arterial occlusive disease, and in particular peripheral arterial occlusive disease (PAOD), is characterized by reduced blood flow through the major blood vessels of the body because of an obstruction or narrowing of the lumen of the aorta and its major branches. Changes in the arterial wall include the accumulation of lipids, calcium, blood components, carbohydrates, and fibrous tissue in the endothelial lining. Arterial occlusive disease, which may be chronic or acute, may affect the celiac, mesenteric, innominate, subclavian, carotid, and vertebral arteries. Arterial disorders that may lead to arterial obstruction include arteriosclerosis obliterans, thromboangiitis obliterans, arterial embolism, and an aneurysm of the lower extremity.

A sudden occlusion usually causes tissue ischemia and death, whereas a gradual blockage allows for the development of collateral vessels. Usually, arterial occlusive diseases are only part of a complex disease syndrome that affects the entire body. Complications include severe ischemia, skin ulceration, gangrene, leg amputation, and sepsis.

Where It Occurs

- Thromboangiitis obliterans, a causative factor for arterial occlusive disease, typically occurs in male smokers between ages 20 and 40.
- Arterial insufficiency usually occurs in individuals over 50 years of age and is more common in men than women.

Signal Symptoms

- Absence of a normally palpable pulse.
- Cold, pale leg or legs.
- Thickened and opaque nails, shiny and atrophic skin, decreased hair growth, dry or fissured heels, and loss of subcutaneous tissue in the digits.

BE SAFE! Check peripheral pulses often and act immediately if they are not palpable.

Diagnostic Tests

Test	What It Tells	Patient Problems/ Nursing Care
Ultrasound arteriography (Doppler ultrasonography)	Reflects the velocity of blood flowing in the underlying vessel, structure, and size	Knowledge deficit: explain procedures.
Segmental arterial pressure monitoring	Simultaneous sphygmomanometer readings of systolic pressure placed on the extremities to measure pressure differences between upper and lower and between like extremities	Knowledge deficit: explain that the test is like having two blood pressures taken at the same time.

Treatment and Nursing Care

Potential Nursing Diagnoses*

Impaired tissue perfusion (peripheral)
Impaired tissue integrity
Knowledge deficit (medications, skin care, postoperative management)
Risk for infection

BE SMART! Bruit over main arteries may indicate an athero-matous plaque.

- Surgery is indicated for patients who have advanced arterial disease or for those with severe pain that impairs activities.
- Aspirin inhibits prostaglandin synthesis, which prevents formation of platelet-aggregating thromboxane A2.
- Anticoagulants prevent extension of a clot and inhibit further clot formation.
- Nursing care should focus on prevention and teaching.

Cardiac Arrhythmias

Cardiac arrhythmias are disturbances in the normal electrical conduction of the heart. They are categorized by the site of origin of the impulse (atrium, atrioventricular junction, or ventricular), heart rate (tachycardia or bradycardia), or mechanism of conduction (block). The etiology of any arrhythmia varies: it may be chemical (electrolyte imbalance), structural (damage to the conduction system), or abnormal automaticity or reentry phenomena. Common causes include myocardial infarction; structural heart changes; electrolyte imbalance; or stimulants such as caffeine, cocaine, and alcohol use.

Where It Occurs

- The incidence of cardiac arrhythmias increases with age.
- Men are more likely than women to have ventricular arrhythmias.
- Approximately 90% of patients who have a myocardial infarction have cardiac arrhythmias.

Signal Symptoms

- Varies with the arrhythmias. Some arrhythmias cause no symptoms, and others life-threatening symptoms.
- Symptoms depend on the perfusion afforded by the arrhythmia; ventricular rhythms may lead to dizziness or loss of consciousness.
- Rapid atrial rhythms may lead to palpitations, chest pain, and/or anxiety.

BE SAFE! Ventricular fibrillation is the most common arrhythmia in cardiac arrest. Begin CPR immediately.

Diagnostic Tests

Test	What It Tells	Patient Problems/ Nursing Care
Electrocardiogram	Documents normal sinus rhythm or suspected arrhythmia; if normal sinus rhythm is found, a Holter can be used to further investigate a possible arrhythmia	Knowledge deficit: explain procedures.
Serum electrolytes	Documents whether electrolyte abnormalities such as potassium and magnesium might contribute to arrhythmias	Knowledge deficit: explain procedures. Patient will need venipuncture.

Treatment and Nursing Care

Potential Nursing Diagnoses*

Ineffective airway clearance
Activity intolerance
Anxiety
Knowledge deficit (medications, reduction of alcohol or cocaine use, stress reduction)

BE SMART! If you notice an arrhythmia on a monitor, always check first that the patient has adequate airway, breathing, and circulation. Electrical interference can sometimes mimic cardiac arrhythmias.

- Varies with the arrhythmia and includes symptomatic treatment of the patient and treatment of the underlying cause.
- Oxygen and lidocaine are often the first treatment modalities used for ventricular tachycardia.
- Place patients on a cardiac monitor.
- Teach patients to avoid stimulants such as caffeine or excessive alcohol use if they are experiencing atrial tachycardia.

Cardiac Catheterization

Cardiac catheterization, insertion of a catheter into the chambers or vessels of the heart, is the standard diagnostic test to evaluate cardiac hemo- dynamics (intracardiac pressure measurements, direct measurements of venous oxygen saturation, and measurement of cardiac output). Most physicians use a percutaneous (through the skin) approach from the femoral, radial, brachial, or axillary artery. Right heart catheterization is usually done percutaneously through the femoral, internal jugular, or subclavian veins.

Usually a left ventriculogram is also completed to assess left ventricular function along with an angiogram of the coronary vessels. The findings help the physician identify healthy areas of the heart that might benefit from coronary artery bypass surgery if it is indicated. Other procedures that might occur during the diagnostic test are atrial pacing, dynamic exercise, and the response to pharmacologic agents.

Where It Occurs

- Indications include determining extent, severity, and location of coronary artery disease; determining left ventricular function; and assessing disorders of the cardiac valves.
- People with uncontrolled hypertension, acute stroke, bleeding disorders, and ventricular arrhythmias are usually considered too at risk to have the procedure.
- Between 2 and 3 million cardiac catheterizations are completed each year in the United States. More men than women have cardiac catheterizations each year, and women tend to have them at an older age. Doctors refer more men than women for the procedure suggesting a possible gender bias.

Signal Symptoms

- Patients are referred for cardiac catheterization when they have signs and symptoms of coronary artery disease, valvular disease, or cardiomyopathy.

BE SAFE! Patients with allergies to radiographic contrast should not have a cardiac catheterization, or they at least need careful assessment and planning before the procedure.

Diagnostic Tests

Test	What It Tells	Patient Problems/ Nursing Care
Complete blood count	Determines if infection or postprocedure bleeding occurred	Knowledge deficit: explain procedures. Patient will need venipuncture.

Treatment and Nursing Care

Potential Nursing Diagnoses*

Ineffective tissue perfusion (peripheral, coronary)
Pain (acute)
Risk for infection
Risk for fluid volume deficit

BE SMART! Coronary angiography is the main strategy to diagnose coronary artery disease and allows the physician to assess the site and extent of abnormalities in the coronary circulation.

- Complications include hypotension, bleeding from the puncture site, heart failure, arrhythmias, chest pain, stroke, infection, allergic reaction, renal failure, and even death.
- Patients need to provide informed consent for the procedure and should understand the risks and benefits.
- Pre- and postprocedural teaching is important.

Cardiac Stent Procedure

A coronary stent, a small tube placed in the coronary arteries to maintain myocardial blood supply in a stenosed or blocker artery, is inserted during a percutaneous coronary intervention similar to a cardiac catheterization. Stents can be made of a variety of materials, such as metal or polymer, and can release, or *elute*, medications. Stents reduce cardiac symptoms such as chest pain and cardiac damage occurring in myocardial infarction. Research has shown that stents may improve survivability following myocardial infarction.

Where It Occurs

- Of the 500,000 deaths from coronary artery disease (CAD) in the United States annually, approximately 160,000 occur before age 65. More than half of these deaths occur in women.
- More than 2 million people worldwide have stents inserted each year.
- African Americans have a higher risk for heart disease than do Whites/European Americans.

Signal Symptoms

- Diaphoresis, clammy skin, nausea and vomiting, and shortness of breath.
- Mild symptoms such as epigastric discomfort.

BE SAFE! Patients are usually placed on medications such as aspirin and clopidogrel/Plavix to reduce the risk for blood clots.

Diagnostic Tests

Test	What It Tells	Patient Problems/ Nursing Care
Intravascular ultrasound (IVUS)	Assesses coronary artery lesion's degree of calcification, size, texture	Knowledge deficit: explain procedures. Patient will need venipuncture.

Treatment and Nursing Care

Potential Nursing Diagnoses*

Ineffective tissue perfusion (peripheral, coronary)
Pain (acute)
Risk for infection
Risk for fluid volume deficit

BE SMART! Stents are foreign bodies and can cause an immune response.

- Complications include hypotension, bleeding from the puncture site, heart failure, arrhythmias, chest pain, stroke, infection, allergic reaction, renal failure, and even death.
- Patients need to provide informed consent for the procedure and should understand the risks and benefits.
- Pre- and postprocedural teaching is important.
- Encourage patients to reduce risk by quitting smoking, monitoring blood pressure and cholesterol levels, reducing weight, getting regular exercise, and reducing stress.

Cardiac Tamponade

Acute cardiac tamponade is a sudden accumulation of fluid in the pericardial sac leading to an increase in the intrapericardial pressure. The pericardial sac surrounds the heart and normally contains only 10 to 20 mL of serous fluid. The sudden accumulation of more fluid (as little as 200 mL of fluid or blood) compresses the heart and coronary arteries, compromising diastolic filling and systolic emptying and diminishing oxygen supply. The result is decreased oxygen delivery and poor tissue perfusion to all organs.

Cardiac tamponade may have any of a variety of etiologies. It can be caused by both blunt and penetrating traumatic injuries and by iatrogenic injuries, such as those associated with removal of epicardial pacing wires and complications after cardiac catheterization and insertion of central venous or pulmonary artery catheters.

Where It Occurs

- Because trauma is the leading cause of death for individuals in the first four decades of life, traumatic tamponade is more common in that age group, whereas the older adult is more likely to have an iatrogenic tamponade.
- Males have higher rates of unintentional injury than do females; in children, cardiac tamponade is more common in boys than in girls with a male-to-female ratio of 7:3.
- Cardiac tamponade related to human immunodeficiency virus infection is more common in young adults, whereas cardiac tamponade due to malignancy or renal failure is more often seen in elderly patients.

- Chest pain, dyspnea, tachycardia, tachypnea.
- Acutely hypovolemia because of blood loss into the pericardial sac; profound cardiac compromise and cardiogenic shock.
- Pericardial friction rub if the two inflamed layers of the pericardium rub against each other.

BE SAFE! Cardiac tamponade is a medical emergency that needs to be managed rapidly.

Diagnostic Tests

Test	What It Tells	Patient Problems/ Nursing Care
Echocardiogram	Echo-free zone anterior to right ventricular wall and posterior to the left ventricular wall; there may also be a decrease in right ventricular chamber size and a right-to-left septal shift during inspiration	Knowledge deficit: explain procedures.

Treatment and Nursing Care

Potential Nursing Diagnoses*

Decreased cardiac output
Ineffective tissue perfusion (cardiopulmonary, peripheral, cerebral)
Pain (acute)
Ineffective breathing pattern

BE SMART! If the patient suffers hypoxia as a result of decreased cardiac output and poor tissue perfusion, oxygen, intubation, and mechanical ventilation may be required.

■ The highest priority is to make sure the patient has adequate airway, breathing, and circulation.

■ Sympathomimetics such as dopamine hydrochloride support blood pressure and cardiac output in emergencies until bleeding is brought under control but are used only if fluid resuscitation is initiated.

Cardiomyopathy

Cardiomyopathy is a chronic or subacute disease process that involves the heart muscle and causes systolic dysfunction or diastolic dysfunction, or both; it most commonly involves the endocardium and occasionally the pericardium. Cardiomyopathy can be classified in several ways. It can be classified as primary when the cause is not known. Secondary cardiomyopathy is a result of some other primary disease process. Cardiomyopathies may also be divided into dilated or nondilated categories.

Three common classifications of cardiomyopathy are dilated, hypertrophic, and restrictive. Dilated cardiomyopathy is the most common and is characterized by ventricular dilation, impaired systolic function, atrial enlargement, and stasis of blood in the left ventricle. This form of cardiomyopathy is progressive and leads to intractable congestive heart failure (CHF) and death in the majority of patients within 5 years.

Hypertrophic cardiomyopathy (HCM), also known as *hypertrophic obstructive cardiomyopathy* or *idiopathic hypertrophic subaortic stenosis*, consists of ventricular hypertrophy, rapid contraction of the left ventricle, and impaired relaxation. It is commonly the result of hypertension or valvular heart disease. The process may go on for years with no or slowly progressive symptoms, or the first sign of the disease may be sudden cardiac death. Although the patient may live a "normal" life, deterioration usually occurs. The third form of cardiomyopathy, restricted cardiomyopathy, is the least common form. Both ventricles become rigid, which distorts the filling phase of the heart. The contraction phase remains normal. The result is that ventricular walls become fibrotic, cardiac filling diminishes, and cardiac output decreases. Restricted cardiomyopathy has a poor prognosis; many patients die within 1 to 2 years after diagnosis.

The etiology of many cases remains a mystery. Ischemic cardiomyopathy is generally considered the most common cause of cardiomyopathy. The major cause of dilated cardiomyopathy is excessive alcohol consumption. Cardiomyopathy may also be caused by amyloidosis, hemochromatosis, metastatic carcinoma affecting the myocardium, fibrosis secondary to radiation, hypertension, vitamin deficiencies, pregnancy, viral or bacterial infection, and immune disorders.

Where It Occurs

- Cardiomyopathy can occur at any age.
- HCM usually occurs in young adults with a family history of the disease.
- Dilated cardiomyopathy, which is twice as common among men as women, occurs most often in middle age.

Signal Symptoms

- Early signs: decreased exercise tolerance, angina, palpitations from arrhythmias such as atrial fibrillation and premature ventricular contractions.
- Later signs: shortness of breath, orthopnea, dyspnea on exertion, peripheral edema.

BE SAFE! Encourage patients to have exercise intolerance worked up by a health provider.

Diagnostic Tests

Test	What It Tells	Patient Problems/ Nursing Care
Echocardiogram: two-dimensional and Doppler	Illustrates impaired systolic and/or diastolic functioning of the heart and differentiates various conditions	Knowledge deficit: explain all procedures.
Cardiac catheterization	Illustrates impaired systolic and/or diastolic functioning of the heart	See Cardiac Catheterization.

Treatment and Nursing Care

Potential Nursing Diagnoses*

Decreased cardiac output

Activity intolerance

Pain (acute)

Ineffective tissue perfusion (coronary, peripheral)

Ineffective breathing pattern

> **BE SMART!** People with late-stage cardiomyopathy may benefit from surgical consultation for procedures such as partial left ventriculectomy or heart transplantation.

- The treatment for cardiomyopathy is palliative rather than curative.
- Angiotensin-converting enzyme (ACE) inhibitors decrease mortality rates in patients with left ventricular dysfunction and reduce readmissions caused by heart failure.
- Digoxin improves contractility and slows the renin-angiotensin response in patients with idiopathic dilated cardiomyopathy.
- In emergencies, treatment involves oxygen, nitrates, and diuretics with ventilator assistance as needed.
- Elevate the head of the patient's bed 30 to 45 degrees to help alleviate dyspnea.
- Teach patient about treatment options, including medications, exercise, diet, and surgical intervention options such as heart transplant.

Coronary Artery Disease

Coronary artery disease (CAD) is the leading cause of death and illness in Western societies and accounts for 20% of all deaths. Atherosclerosis is the most common cause of CAD and is linked to many risk factors—primarily elevated serum cholesterol levels, elevated blood pressure, and cigarette smoking. A number of conditions result from CAD, including angina, congestive heart failure, myocardial infarction, and sudden cardiac death. CAD results when decreased blood flow through the coronary arteries causes inadequate delivery of oxygen and nutrients to the myocardium. The lumens of the coronary arteries become narrowed from either fatty fibrous plaques or calcium plaque deposits, thus reducing blood flow to the myocardium, which can lead to chest pain or even myocardial infarction (MI) and sudden cardiac death.

Plaque buildup in the coronary arteries is a result of arteriosclerosis, defined as thickening of the arterial walls' inner aspect and a loss of elasticity. Arterial walls may develop calcifications, which diminish the ability of the vessels to transport blood adequately. Atherosclerosis, the most common form of arteriosclerosis, produces yellowish plaques made up mostly of cholesterol and lipids that line the inner arterial wall. The process of atherosclerosis may be initiated by damage to the arterial endothelium. Plaque accumulation reduces the inner arterial lumen and leads to wall thickening, calcification, and reduced blood supply. Aging results in increased streaking of fatty substances and fibrous change in the arteries.

Where It Occurs

- Of the 500,000 deaths from CAD in the United States annually, approximately 160,000 occur before age 65. More than half of these occur in women.
- Native Americans have a higher risk for heart disease than do whites, although Hispanics have the lowest risk for heart disease compared with all these groups.
- Asian Indians living in the United States exhibit two to three times higher prevalence of CAD than whites.
- Genetic and nonmodifiable risk factors: sex, age, family history with heart disease in the father or a brother before age 55 or the mother or a sister before age 65.
- Modifiable risk factors: elevated cholesterol, tobacco use, diabetes mellitus, exposure to air pollution, obesity, lack of exercise, elevated blood pressure, stress, depression.

Signal Symptoms

- Many people are asymptomatic; physical examination may reveal nothing abnormal.
- Chest pain and/or shortness of breath on exertion, referred (jaw, back, or arm) pain, dizziness, palpitations, diaphoresis.

■ Late: evidence of flat or slightly raised yellowish tumors, most frequently found on the upper and lower lids (xanthelasma), or flat, slightly elevated, soft, rounded plaques or nodules, usually on the eyelids (xanthoma).

BE SAFE! Labored breathing, pallor, and profuse sweating accompanied by chest pain suggest myocardial infarction.

Diagnostic Tests: See also Cardiac Catheterization

Test	What It Tells	Patient Problems/ Nursing Care
Lipid profile	Elevated cholesterol levels are associated with CAD	Knowledge deficit: explain procedures. Patient will need venipuncture.
Electrocardiogram (ECG)	Changes in the electrical activity of the heart are associated with cardiac ischemia, injury, or necrosis	Knowledge deficit: explain procedures.
Computed tomography angiography	May show presence of a plaque in asymptomatic patients	Knowledge deficit: explain procedures.

Treatment and Nursing Care

Potential Nursing Diagnoses*

Altered tissue perfusion (cardiopulmonary)
Pain (acute)
Ineffective breathing pattern
Activity intolerance
Anxiety
Knowledge deficit (prevention, risk factors, medications, treatment options, rest/activity, stress reduction, diet)

BE SMART! Teach the patient to modify risk factors using evidence-based practice protocols.

- Several invasive but nonsurgical procedures can be used to manage CAD, including balloon catheter angioplasty and stenting.
- Many new biological (C-reactive protein, lipoprotein(a), fibrinogen, homocysteine) and genetic markers are being used to determine the presence of CAD or the risk for CAD.
- Aspirin reduces incidence of myocardial infarction by preventing clots.
- Nitrates and other antianginal agents increase coronary artery blood flow through vasodilation.
- Standard treatment also often includes beta blockers, statins, calcium channel blockers, and ranolazine.
- During episodes of chest pain, encourage complete rest and allay the patient's anxiety by remaining close at hand.
- Patient education is the cornerstone of managing CAD. A wealth of information is available on education for diet, physical activity, medications, modifying risk, smoking cessation, sensible alcohol use, and treatment options.

Cor Pulmonale

Cor pulmonale is right-sided hypertrophy of the heart caused by a primary disorder of the respiratory system, pulmonary hypertension. Cor pulmonale causes approximately 5% to 7% of all types of heart disease in adults, and chronic obstructive pulmonary disease (COPD) due to chronic bronchitis or emphysema is the causative factor in more than 50% of people with cor pulmonale. It causes increases in pulmonary resistance, and as the right side of the heart works harder, the right ventricle hypertrophies. An increase in pulmonary vascular resistance is the result of anatomic reduction of the pulmonary vascular bed, pulmonary vasoconstriction, or abnormalities of ventilatory mechanics.

Cor pulmonale is produced by a number of other pulmonary and pulmonary vascular disorders. Acute cor pulmonale is most commonly caused by a massive pulmonary embolism. In contrast, it generally has a slow, progressive course, but rapidly deteriorating cor pulmonale with life-threatening complications can occur.

Where It Occurs

- Middle-aged to elderly men are more likely to experience cor pulmonale, but incidence in women is increasing.
- In children, cor pulmonale is likely to be a complication of cystic fibrosis, hemosiderosis, upper airway obstruction, scleroderma, extensive bronchiectasis, neurological diseases that affect the respiratory muscles, or abnormalities of the respiratory control center.

Signal Symptoms

- Fatigue, tachycardia, shortness of breath at rest that increases to acute dyspnea on exertion, cough, peripheral edema.
- The use of accessory muscles in breathing.
- Chest pain, hemoptysis, dizziness, syncope.
- Late signs: anorexia, right-upper-quadrant abdominal pain, jaundice. Hoarseness.

BE SAFE! Place the patient on oxygen to ensure adequate oxygen delivery to the tissues.

Diagnostic Tests: See also Cardiac Catheterization

Test	What It Tells	Patient Problems/ Nursing Care
Chest x-rays	Enlarged right ventricle and pulmonary artery; may show pneumonia	Knowledge deficit: explain procedures.
Electrocardiogram (ECG)	Changes in cardiac conduction due to right-sided hypertrophy	Knowledge deficit: explain procedures.

Treatment and Nursing Care

Potential Nursing Diagnoses*

Decreased cardiac output
Ineffective breathing pattern

Sell your books at
sellbackyourBook.com!
Go to sellbackyourBook.com
and get an instant price
quote. We even pay the
shipping - see what your old
books are worth today!

Inspected By: MaElena_Aguilar

00064355114

0006435 **5114** c-2
S-1

Pain (acute)

Ineffective tissue perfusion (cerebral, peripheral)

Anxiety

> **BE SMART!** Manage pulmonary infections immediately so that oxygenation is not further compromised.

- Long-term management of chronic cor pulmonale includes oxygen, diuretics, vasodilators, cardiac inotropes, bronchodilators, anticoagulants.
- The patient with an acute exacerbation may require mechanical ventilation and oxygenation.
- Calcium channel blockers lower pulmonary pressures.
- Bronchodilators relieve bronchospasm.
- In an emergency to support left ventricular function, patients may receive fluid loading and epinephrine to assist peripheral perfusion.
- Provide skin care to the patient on bedrest.
- Teach patients to control their anxiety, which affects their breathlessness and fear.

Deep Vein Thrombosis

Thrombophlebitis, inflammation of a vein with an associated blood clot (thrombus), typically occurs in the veins of the lower extremities when fibrin and platelets accumulate at areas of stasis or turbulence near venous valves. Venous stasis, hypercoagulability, and vascular injury are major causes of thrombophlebitis. Deep vein thrombophlebitis (deep vein thrombosis [DVT]) occurs more than 90% of the time in small veins, such as the lesser saphenous, or in large veins, such as the femoral and popliteal. DVT and its possible consequence, pulmonary embolism, are the leading causes of preventable mortality in hospitalized patients in the United States.

DVT is potentially more serious than thrombosis of the superficial veins because the deep veins carry approximately 90% of the blood flow as it leaves the lower extremities. Once a thrombus begins to move, it becomes an embolus (a detached intravascular mass carried by the blood). If it reaches the lungs, a pulmonary embolus, it is potentially fatal. Risk factors include immobility, dehydration, venous stasis, and increased blood viscosity. The primary life-threatening complication is pulmonary embolism.

Where It Occurs

- Young women and the elderly are more likely than adult men to develop thrombophlebitis because young adult women may have many risk factors (pregnancy, oral contraceptives, smoking, obesity).
- The elderly person's increased tendency for platelet aggregation and elevated fibrinogen levels increases risk.

Signal Symptoms

- Pain, swelling.
- Redness, warmth, and discoloration when compared with the contralateral limb.
- Superficial veins over the area may be distended.

BE SAFE! Teach patients at risk for thrombophlebitis to remain well hydrated and keep extremities moving during long periods of sitting, such as on plane rides.

Diagnostic Tests

Test	What It Tells	Patient Problems/ Nursing Case
D-dimer, measured by latex agglutination or by an enzyme-linked immunosorbent assay test	D-dimer fragments are present in a fresh fibrin clot, and levels are elevated for 7 days when clots form	Knowledge deficit: explain procedures. Patient will need venipuncture.
Doppler ultrasound; duplex Doppler venous scanning	Records sound waves reflected from moving red blood cells in arteries and veins and demonstrates diminished flow	Knowledge deficit: explain procedures.

Treatment and Nursing Care

Potential Nursing Diagnoses*

Ineffective tissue perfusion (peripheral)
Pain (acute)
Activity intolerance
Anxiety

> **BE SMART!** Patients on anticoagulants must be taught to watch for signs and symptoms of excessive bleeding or hemorrhage risk.

- Most patients who develop thrombophlebitis are placed on bedrest with extremity elevation to avoid dislodging the thrombus.
- Fibrinolytic agents break down the blood clot for deep vein thrombosis.
- Low-molecular-weight heparin is the treatment of choice for superficial venous thrombosis.
- Anticoagulants reduce further formation of clots.
- Aspirin and NSAIDs are useful to relieve pain.
- The most important nursing interventions focus on prevention, use of graduated support stockings, and adequate hydration.

Fat Embolism

An embolism is any undissolved mass that travels in the circulation and occludes a blood vessel. A fat embolism, which is an unusual complication from a traumatic injury, occurs when fat droplets enter the circulation and lodge in small vessels and capillaries, particularly in the lung and brain. Two theories exist that explain the pathophysiology of fat emboli: the mechanical theory and the biochemical theory. The mechanical theory states that trauma disrupts fat cells and tears veins in the bone marrow at the site of a fracture. Fat droplets enter the circulation because of increased pressure of the interstitium at the area of injury. The biochemical theory states that a stress-related release of catecholamines after trauma mobilizes fat molecules from a tissue. These molecules group into fat droplets and eventually obstruct the circulation. In addition, free fatty acids destroy pulmonary endothelium, increase capillary permeability in the lungs, and lead to pulmonary edema.

The result of either theory is the accumulation of fat droplets that are too large to pass easily through small capillaries, where they lodge and break apart into fatty acids, which are toxic to lung tissues, the capillary endothelium, and surfactant. Pulmonary hypertension, alveolar collapse, and even noncardiac pulmonary edema follow.

Where It Occurs

- Trauma patients under age 30; males are more likely than females to have a significant traumatic injury.
- Patients receiving lipid infusions.
- Severe burns, massive soft tissue injury, bone marrow biopsy, liposuction, acute panceratitis.

Signal Symptoms

- Shortness of breath, rapid heart and respiratory rate, and fever.
- Petechiae, a classic sign that appears 1 to 2 days after injury in more than half of patients with fat embolism, usually occurs on the upper trunk and beneath the arms.
- Agitation, delirium, seizures.

BE SAFE! Note that neurological changes usually occur 6 to 12 hours before respiratory system changes and rarely without impending respiratory involvement.

Diagnostic Tests

Test	What It Tells	Patient Problems/ Nursing Care
Platelet count	Decreased count because platelets are used up in the clotting process	Knowledge deficit: explain procedures. Patient will need venipuncture.
Partial pressure of oxygen in the blood (Pao_2)	Hypoxemia occurs because of problems with ventilation and perfusion due to obstruction of pulmonary circulation	Knowledge deficit: explain procedures. Patient will need arterial puncture. Warn patient that the procedure is painful.

Potential Nursing Diagnoses*

Ineffective airway clearance
Ineffective breathing pattern
Impaired skin integrity
Confusion, acute

BE SMART! Be prepared to assist with endotracheal intubation if the patient's airway becomes compromised.

- Management of the patient almost always requires support of the patient's airway and breathing with supplemental oxygen and possibly endotracheal intubation and mechanical ventilation.
- The nurse and trauma surgeon or orthopedist work together to prevent fat emboli whenever possible by encouraging adequate gas exchange.
- Corticosteroids decrease inflammatory response of pulmonary capillaries and stabilize lysosomal and capillary membranes.
- The highest priority is maintaining airway, breathing, and circulation.

Heart Failure

Heart failure (HF) occurs when the heart is unable to pump sufficient blood to meet the metabolic needs of the body. It is the most common nonfatal consequence of cardiovascular disorders and is the only major heart disease that is increasing significantly throughout the world. The result of inadequate cardiac output (CO) is poor organ perfusion and vascular congestion in the pulmonary or systemic circulation.

HF may be described as backward or forward failure, high- or low-output failure, or right- or left-sided failure. HF may result from a number of causes that affect preload (venous return), afterload (impedance the heart has to overcome to eject its volume), or contractility.

The primary alterations that occur in HF are due to the myocardial response to increased wall stress as the heart works hard to move blood forward. This leads to myocyte (heart muscle cells) hypertrophy, death, and regeneration. The heart can show myocardial hypertrophy with or without dilatation and activation of neurohumoral systems (norepinephrine, epinephrine, and the sympathetic nervous system, renin-angiotensin-aldosterone system, endothelin-1 [ET-1], and vasopressin) that help maintain tissue perfusion but generally cause vasoconstriction. Primary causes include coronary artery disease and myocardial infarction, high blood pressure, diabetes mellitus, arrhythmias, valvular heart disease, myocarditis.

Where It Occurs

■ Elderly people are much more prone to HF because of chronic hypertension, coronary artery disease, myocardial infarction, chronic ischemia, or valve disease, all of which occur more frequently in the elderly population.
■ As compared with whites, the incidence and prevalence of HF are higher in African Americans, Hispanic/Latinos, and Native Americans.
■ Men and women develop HF in the same proportion, but women develop it later in life, are more likely to have HF-associated depression, and have more severe symptoms even while living longer.

Signal Symptoms

■ Tachycardia, edema, activity intolerance, fatigue, orthopnea, dyspnea at rest, nocturnal dyspnea.
■ Mental confusion, anxiety, or irritability caused by hypoxia.
■ Pale or cyanotic, cool, clammy skin.

BE SAFE! Acute pulmonary edema is a life-threatening condition associated with HF. Edema reduction and breathing support are critical.

Diagnostic Tests

Test	What It Tells	Patient Problems/ Nursing Care
Echocardiography (ECHO)	Demonstrates depressed cardiac output, evidence of cardiomegaly	Knowledge deficit: explain procedures.
Multigated blood pool imaging	Demonstrates alterations in cardiac output and ejection fraction, often decreased	Knowledge deficit: explain procedures.

Potential Nursing Diagnoses*

Decreased cardiac output
Ineffective tissue perfusion (coronary, peripheral)
Activity intolerance
Anxiety
Ineffective breathing pattern

> **BE SMART!** Patient education is critical on subjects such as self-management, medications, physical activity, treatment options, and nutrition.

- The general principle for management is treatment of any precipitating causes.
- If the elevated preload is caused by valvular regurgitation, the patient may require corrective surgery. Heart transplant is available for some patients depending on presentation and health history.
- Drug therapy can be complex and include drugs blocking the beta-adrenergic system (metoprolol and carvedilol); use of angiotensin-converting enzyme inhibitors (ACEIs), angiotensin receptor blockers (ARBs), loop and thiazide diuretics, aldosterone antagonists, and digoxin.
- End-stage patients may need intravenous inotropes, vasodilators to reduce vasoconstriction, thereby reducing afterload and enhancing myocardial performance and decreasing preload and ventricular filling pressures.
- Diuretics are used for patients with volume overload.
- To control symptoms, provide ongoing monitoring throughout the acute phases of the patient's disease.
- Toward the end of life, palliative care is important.

Hypertension

Hypertension, one of the globe's most common diseases, is a persistent or intermittent elevation of systolic arterial blood pressure above 140 mm Hg or diastolic pressure above 90 mm Hg. Hypertension is classified by three types: Primary (essential) accounts for over 90% of cases and is often referred to as *idiopathic* because the underlying cause is not known. This type has an insidious onset with few, if any, symptoms, so it is often not recognized until complications occur.

Secondary hypertension results from a number of conditions that impair blood pressure regulation, and this type accounts for only 5% to 8% of all cases of hypertension. A severe or accelerating form of hypertension, malignant hypertension, results from either type and can cause blood pressures as high as 240/150 mm Hg, possibly leading to coma and death. Untreated, hypertension can cause major complications.

At least 30% of people with hypertension are undiagnosed. Risk factors include elevated cholesterol, type 1 and type 2 diabetes, oral contraceptives, illicit drug use such as cocaine, and alcohol and/or tobacco use. Obesity and high-salt diet are also associated with hypertension.

Where It Occurs

- Malignant hypertension affects men more often than women, with the average age at diagnosis being 40 years. Hypertension increases with age.
- African Americans and elderly people are most prone to hypertension and its complications.
- Mexican Americans and Native Americans have lower blood pressure than non-Hispanic whites and African Americans.

Signal Symptoms

- The patient may appear symptom free in early stages, although flushing of the face may be present.
- An atrial gallop (S_4) heart sound, ocular changes, headache, migraines, dizziness, blurred vision, chest pain.
- Secondary causes of hypertension include thyroid or renal disease, anemia, and pheochromocytoma.

BE SAFE! Regular blood pressure screening is critical to improve the pubic health.

Diagnostic Tests

Test	What It Tells	Patient Problems/ Nursing Care
Blood urea nitrogen	May be elevated, indicating presence of renal dysfunction or fluid imbalances	Knowledge deficit: explain procedures. Patient will need venipuncture.
Serum creatinine	Indicates renal dysfunction is present as a complication of hypertension	Knowledge deficit: explain procedures. Patient will need venipuncture.

Treatment and Nursing Care

Potential Nursing Diagnoses*

Knowledge deficit (medications, diet, smoking cessation, alcohol use, chronic disease management)
Pain (acute)
Anxiety
Ineffective coping

> **BE SMART!** For an accurate blood pressure measurement, allow the patient to relax quietly before the measurement.

- The long-term goal of care is to limit organ damage.
- The primary goal is to reduce the blood pressure to less than 140/90 mm Hg.
- Beta-adrenergic antagonists inhibit effects of catecholamines that decrease renin and cause resetting of baroreceptors to accept a lower level of blood pressure.
- Educate the patient about the pathophysiology and treatment of hypertension.

Infective Endocarditis

Infective endocarditis (IE) is an inflammatory process that typically affects a deformed or previously damaged valve, which is usually the focus of the infection. Typically, endocarditis occurs when an invading organism enters the bloodstream and attaches to the leaflets of the valves or the endocardium. Bacteria multiply and sometimes form a projection of tissue that includes bacteria, fibrin, red blood cells, and white blood cells on the valves of the heart. This clump of material, called vegetation, may eventually cover the entire valve surface, leading to ulceration and tissue necrosis. Vegetation may even extend to the chordae tendineae, causing them to rupture and the valve to become incompetent.

IE can occur as an acute or a subacute condition. Generally, acute IE is a rapidly progressing infection, whereas subacute IE progresses more slowly. Acute endocarditis usually occurs on a normal heart valve and is rapidly destructive and fatal in 6 weeks if it is left untreated. Subacute endocarditis usually occurs in a heart already damaged by congenital or acquired heart disease, on damaged valves, and takes up to a year to cause death if it is left untreated. Since the 1960s, the most common causes of IE are nosocomial infections from IV catheters, IV drug abuse, pacemaker insertion, and prosthetic valve endocarditis.

Where It Occurs

- Males are affected three times more than females.
- Up to half of the cases occur in people older than 60 years.
- Men over age 45 are at highest risk.

Signal Symptoms

- The patient appears acutely ill, but symptoms vary widely.
- Temperature elevation, such as warm skin, dry mucous membranes, and alternating chills and diaphoresis; night sweats; dyspnea; cough; chest pain.
- Approximately 95% of those with subacute IE have a heart murmur (most commonly mitral and aortic regurgitation murmurs), which is typically absent in patients with acute IE.

BE SAFE! Watch for accompanying signs of heart failure, including shortness of breath, peripheral edema, activity intolerance, cough.

Diagnostic Tests

Test	What It Tells	Patient Problems/ Nursing Care
Blood cultures and sensitivities (three to five sets of cultures over 24 hr)	Positive for microorganisms in 90% of patients	Knowledge deficit: explain procedures. Patient will need venipuncture.

Treatment and Nursing Care

Potential Nursing Diagnoses*

Risk for infection
Hyperthermia
Risk for injury
Knowledge deficit (medications, physical activity)

BE SMART! IV drug users often present with cough, dyspnea, and chest pain, particularly if they have valvular involvement.

- For persons at high risk for contracting IE, most physicians prescribe antibiotic therapy to prevent episodes of bacteremia before, during, and after invasive procedures.
- Oxygen and antibiotic therapy are essential. Penicillin G treats penicillin-susceptible streptococcal infections in subacute bacterial endocarditis. Oxacillin treats acute bacterial endocarditis.
- During the acute phase of the disease, provide adequate rest by assisting the patient with daily hygiene.
- Patient teaching is important so that patient knows prevention strategies and to take all antibiotics as prescribed.

Myocardial Infarction

Myocardial infarction (MI) is irreversible myocardial tissue death. It occurs because of absent or diminished blood supply. Infarctions may occur for a variety of reasons, but coronary thrombosis of a coronary artery narrowed with an atherosclerotic plaque is the most common cause. When myocardial tissue is deprived of oxygenated blood supply for a period of time, an area of myocardial necrosis develops; this necrosis is surrounded by injured and ischemic tissue.

Infarctions may be classified according to myocardial thickness and the location of affected tissue. Although the majority of MIs occur in the left ventricle, more right ventricular involvement is being recognized. Left ventricular infarctions are classified as inferior (diaphragmatic), anterior, and posterior. Right ventricular infarctions are usually not differentiated by a specific location. Complications include arrhythmias, heart failure, cardiac rupture, cardiogenic shock. Risk factors include lack of physical activity, cigarette smoking, obesity and overweight, stress, alcohol misuse, and conditions such as hypertension and diabetes mellitus.

Where It Occurs

■ The risk of MI increases with age, and it occurs most commonly in people older than 45 years.
■ MI is the single largest cause of death among American men and women, including white, African American, and Hispanic/Latino populations.
■ There is a genetic predisposition to acute coronary syndrome.

Signal Symptoms

■ Chest pain radiating to arm, chin, neck, or back; may have no pain but report epigastric discomfort.
■ Diaphoresis, clammy skin, nausea, and vomiting.
■ Anxiety, dizziness, cough, shortness of breath.

BE SAFE! Epigastric discomfort may indicate MI; not all patients exhibit the classic signs of radiating chest pain, nausea, and diaphoresis.

Diagnostic Tests

Test	What It Tells	Patient Problems/ Nursing Care
Cardiac troponin I (cTnI); cardiac troponin T (cTnT)	Cardiac troponin levels have the highest sensitivity and specificity in detecting MI and are used to differentiate between angina and MI	Knowledge deficit: explain procedures. Patient will need venipuncture.
Electrocardiogram (ECG)	Demonstrates abnormal electrical conduction system adversely affected by myocardial ischemia and necrosis	Knowledge deficit: explain procedures.

Treatment and Nursing Care

Potential Nursing Diagnoses*

Altered tissue perfusion (cardiopulmonary)

Pain (acute)

Risk for decreased cardiac output

Anxiety

Knowledge deficit (treatment options, diagnostic tests, medications, stress and lifestyle changes)

BE SMART! Administer oxygen immediately and have patient rest to conserve oxygen consumption.

■ The physician usually prescribes oxygen therapy.

■ A cardiac catheterization may be performed when the patient's condition is stable to identify the areas of blockage in the coronary arteries and to assist in determining treatment.

■ Antiplatelet therapy prevents formation of thrombus.

■ Recombinant tissue plasminogen activator (alteplase, rt-PA) is used as a thrombolytic agent.

- Other medications include angiotensin-converting enzyme inhibitors, beta blockers, calcium channel blockers, nitroglycerine, and NSAIDs.
- The focus of treatment is to control pain and related symptoms, to reduce myocardial oxygen consumption during myocardial healing, and to provide patient/family education.

Myocarditis

Myocarditis describes the infiltration of myocardial cells by various forms of bacteria or viruses that damage the myocardium by inciting an inflammatory response and myocyte necrosis. Many people are asymptomatic or have symptoms that may not be attributed to myocarditis. Myocarditis results in white blood cell (WBC) infiltration and necrosis of myocytes (heart muscle cells).

Myocarditis generally occurs as a result of an infectious agent, but it also can be caused by radiation or other toxic physical agents, such as lead.

Where It Occurs

- Males are slightly more affected than females.
- In the United States, myocarditis most typically occurs in the fifth decade of life.

Signal Symptoms

- Fatigue, dyspnea on exertion, activity intolerance, myalgias, fever.
- Pleuritic pain; sharp precordial chest pain.
- Anorexia, weight loss.
- Signs of overt heart failure: edema, shortness of breath, cyanosis, hypotension.

BE SAFE! Begin antibiotics and antivirals early to give the patient the best possible opportunity to recover cardiac function.

Diagnostic Tests

Test	What It Tells	Patient Problems/ Nursing Care
Cardiac troponin I	Elevated result is a sign of inflammation and myocyte necrosis	Knowledge deficit: explain procedures. Patient will need venipuncture.
Endomyocardial biopsy	Presence of abnormal numbers of lymphocytes and degeneration of muscle fibers illustrate the damage to myocytes caused by a virus	Knowledge deficit: explain procedures.

Treatment and Nursing Care

Potential Nursing Diagnoses*

Pain (acute)
Activity intolerance
Hyperthermia
Fatigue
Ineffective breathing pattern

BE SMART! Medication therapy can be complicated. Make sure to explain the rationale, dosage, and side effects of all medications.

- The primary goal of treatment of myocarditis is to eliminate the underlying cause.
- Antibiotics are prescribed to kill pathogens.
- Medications may be used to manage arrhythmias and signs of cardiac failure: angiotensin-converting enzymes, beta blockers, calcium channel blockers, loop diuretics, cardiac glycosides.
- In addition to any prescribed analgesics, nurses should assist the patient with pain management by teaching relaxation techniques, guided imagery, and distractions.
- Nursing care should focus on maximizing oxygen delivery and minimizing oxygen consumption.

Pericarditis

Pericarditis is an inflammation of the pericardium, which is the membranous sac that encloses the heart and great vessels. The inflammatory response causes an accumulation of leukocytes, platelets, fibrin, and fluid between the parietal and visceral layers of the pericardial sac, producing a variety of symptoms, depending on the amount of fluid accumulation, how quickly it accumulates, and whether the inflammation resolves after the acute phase or becomes chronic.

An acute pericardial effusion is caused by an accumulation of fluid in the pericardial sac. The fluid accumulation interferes with cardiac function by compressing the cardiac chambers. Chronic constrictive pericarditis usually begins as an acute inflammatory pericarditis and progresses over time to a chronic, constrictive form because of pericardial thickening and stiffening. The thickened, scarred pericardium becomes nondistensible and decreases diastolic filling of the cardiac chambers and cardiac output. Chronic pericardial effusion is a gradual accumulation of fluid in the pericardial sac. The pericardium is slowly stretched and can accommodate more than 1 liter of fluid at a time. Complications include acute cardiac tamponade.

Where It Occurs

- Idiopathic (viral) inflammatory pericarditis occurs more frequently in adults than in children and is more common in men than in women.
- Tuberculous (bacterial) pericarditis occurs most often in children and in immunosuppressed patients.
- Occurs in people with autoimmune disease such as rheumatoid arthritis and systemic lupus erythematosus.
- Occurs in people with malignant disease and renal failure.

Signal Symptoms

- Precordial or retrosternal chest pain; referred pain to the left arm and shoulder or chin.
- Palpitations, hypotension, pulsus paradoxus, neck vein distention.
- Low-grade fever, dyspnea, tachypnea, cough.

BE SAFE! Pericarditis must be treated promptly so that the underlying cause can be treated (cancer, injury, autoimmune disease, renal failure).

Test	What It Tells	Patient Problems/ Nursing Care
Limited echocardiography	Illustrates accumulation of fluid in the pericardial space	Knowledge deficit: explain procedures.
Electrocardiogram	Demonstrates pericardial thickening and diminished diastolic filling	Knowledge deficit: explain procedures.

Treatment and Nursing Care

Potential Nursing Diagnoses*

Pain (acute)
Ineffective tissue perfusion (cardiopulmonary)
Risk for injury
Risk for infection
Anxiety
Ineffective breathing pattern

> **BE SMART!** People with autoimmune disease are at risk for pericarditis and are often on NSAIDs that can cause bleeding because of their antiplatelet function.

- Pericarditis is treated by correcting the underlying cause.
- NSAIDs reduce pain and inflammation.
- Pericardiocentesis allows for fluid to be removed from the pericardial sac.
- Teach patient how to recognize signs and symptoms, side effects of medications, and the need for emergency care when symptoms occur.

Pulmonary Embolism

Pulmonary embolism (PE) is a potentially life-threatening condition in which a free-flowing blood clot (embolism) becomes lodged within the pulmonary vasculature. A PE usually occurs when a thrombus in the deep veins of the lower extremities loosens or dislodges and begins to move in the bloodstream. When an embolism becomes lodged within a pulmonary vessel, platelets accumulate around the thrombus and trigger the release of potent vasoactive substances. The pulmonary vasculature constricts, which leads to an increased pulmonary vascular resistance, increased pulmonary arterial pressure, and increased right ventricular workload. Blood flow abnormalities result in a ventilation/perfusion mismatch that is initially dead-space ventilation (ventilation with no perfusion).

As atelectasis occurs, shunting (perfusion without ventilation of the alveolus) results. If the right side of the heart (accustomed to pumping out against a relatively low-resistance pulmonary circuit) cannot empty its volume against the increased pulmonary vascular resistance, right-sided heart failure occurs. Ultimately, cardiac function may deteriorate with decreased cardiac output, decreased systemic blood flow, and shock.

Where It Occurs

- PE in children is associated with cardiac conditions and coagulopathic diseases such as sickle cell anemia and cancer.
- Young women are at risk for PE during pregnancy or while they take high-estrogen-content birth control pills.
- Overall men are more at risk than women across the life span, and African Americans are more at risk than other populations.
- More common in the last three decades of life than during younger years.

Signal Symptoms

- Severe shortness of breath, diaphoresis, weakness, anxiety, tachycardia.
- Rales, fever, symptoms suggesting thrombophlebitis (leg swelling, pain, warmth, redness), leg edema.
- Adventitious heart sounds such as murmurs and gallops.
- Chest pain, syncope, and chest splinting, hemoptysis.

BE SAFE! The first few hours are critical for a patient with PE, who needs emergency care immediately.

Diagnostic Tests

Test	What It Tells	Patient Problems/ Nursing Care
Arterial blood gases	Poor gas exchange and shunting leads to hypoxemia	Knowledge deficit: explain all procedures. Patient will need arterial puncture: explain that procedure is painful.
High-resolution multidetector computed tomographic angiography	Can detect obstruction in blood flow in small arteries and veins caused by a clot	Knowledge deficit: explain all procedures.

Treatment and Nursing Care

Potential Nursing Diagnoses*

Impaired gas exchange
Pain (acute)
Anxiety
Ineffective breathing pattern
Risk for injury
Fluid volume deficit

BE SMART! Although it is rare, severe cases of PE that are unresponsive to anticoagulant or thrombolytic therapy may require surgery.

- The patient's airway, breathing, and circulation (ABCs) must be maintained.
- Thrombolytic agents break down clots previously formed and hasten resolution of clots.
- Anticoagulants, such as IV heparin and Coumadin, reduce further formation of clots.
- Prevention: further thrombus formation, hypercoagulation, dehydration.
- Teach patient lifestyle changes, adequate hydration, use and dose of all medications, physical activity tolerance.

Thrombophlebitis

Thrombophlebitis, inflammation of a vein with an associated blood clot (thrombus), typically occurs in the veins of the lower extremities when fibrin and platelets accumulate at areas of stasis or turbulence near venous valves. Deep vein thrombophlebitis (deep vein thrombosis [DVT]) occurs more than 90% of the time in small veins, such as the lesser saphenous, or in large veins, such as the femoral and popliteal.

Venous stasis, hypercoagulability, and vascular injury are major causes of thrombophlebitis. DVT is potentially more serious than thrombosis of the superficial veins because the deep veins carry approximately 90% of the blood flow as it leaves the lower extremities. Once a thrombus begins to move, it becomes an embolus (a detached intravascular mass carried by the blood). If it reaches the lungs, a pulmonary embolus, it is potentially fatal.

Where It Occurs

- Young women and the elderly are more likely than adult men to develop thrombophlebitis because young adult women may have many risk factors (pregnancy, oral contraceptives, smoking, obesity).
- The elderly person's increased tendency for platelet aggregation and elevated fibrinogen levels increases risk.

Signal Symptoms

- DVT: redness, warmth, swelling, pain, and discoloration on affected limb.
- Superficial vein thrombosis: may be asymptomatic; pain, redness, induration, and swelling.

BE SAFE! Note the presence of calf pain with dorsiflexion of the foot of the affected extremity, which is a positive Homans sign. This is one sign of thrombophlebitis.

Diagnostic Tests

Test	What It Tells	Patient Problems/ Nursing Care
D-dimer, measured by latex agglutination or by an enzyme-linked immunosorbent assay test	D-dimer fragments are present in a fresh fibrin clot, and levels are elevated for 7 days when clots form	Knowledge deficit: explain procedures. Patient will need venipuncture.
Doppler ultrasound; duplex Doppler venous scanning	Records sound waves reflected from moving red blood cells in arteries and veins	Knowledge deficit: explain procedures.

Treatment and Nursing Care

Potential Nursing Diagnoses*

Ineffective tissue perfusion (peripheral)
Pain (acute)
Impaired physical mobility
Impaired tissue integrity

BE SMART! Initiate strategies to have patient remain immobile and to rest until risk of embolus decreases.

- To prevent thrombus formation, most physicians prescribe compression of the legs by graduated compression stockings to reduce venous stasis in low-risk general surgical patients.
- Most patients who develop thrombophlebitis are placed on bedrest with extremity elevation to avoid dislodging the thrombus.
- Fibrinolytic agents break down the blood clot for deep vein (but usually not superficial vein) thrombosis.
- Anticoagulants, such as IV heparin, reduce further formation of clots.
- Teach patient strategies to prevent thrombophlebitis: avoid long period of standing or sitting, maintain good hydration, wear support stockings.

Valvular Heart Disease

Valvular heart disease describes cardiac dysfunction that results from structural or functional abnormalities of one or more valves. There are two major types of diseased valves: valvular stenosis, in which the flow of blood from one chamber to the next is impeded, and valvular insufficiency or regurgitation, in which blood leaks back into the chamber from which blood is being pumped.

Valvular heart disease includes mitral stenosis, mitral regurgitation, mitral valve prolapse, aortic stenosis, aortic regurgitation, tricuspid stenosis, and tricuspid regurgitation. With valvular stenosis, the valve orifice's opening narrows and the valve leaflets become fused together in such a way that the valve cannot open freely. With valvular regurgitation, the valve cannot close completely, resulting in blood flowing backward through the opening.

Causes include rheumatic fever, congenital malformations, valvular calcification, and arthrosclerosis.

Where It Occurs

- Mitral stenosis and regurgitation occur more commonly in women; usually found before age 45.
- Mitral insufficiency is more common in women; peaks at age 30, associated with a low body mass index.
- Aortic stenosis from congenital malformations usually occurs before age 30; more common in men.
- Aortic insufficiency usually occurs after age 40 and is more common in men than in women.

Signal Symptoms

- Mitral stenosis: signs of right-sided heart failure: neck vein distention, edema, orthopnea, tachypnea, fatigue, malaise, exercise intolerance.
- Mitral insufficiency: systolic murmur, rales, enlarged liver, jugular vein distention.
- Aortic stenosis: chest pain, syncope, labored breathing on exertion, systolic murmur.
- Aortic insufficiency: apical pulsation, diastolic murmur, rales, widened pulse pressure, tachycardia, labored breathing on exertion.

BE SAFE! Until the decision is made for surgery, conserve the patient's energy with rest.

Diagnostic Tests

Test	What It Tells	Patient Problems/ Nursing Care
Chest x-ray	Illustrates congestion, enlargement, or calcification of cardiac structures related to disease	Knowledge deficit: explain all procedures.
Electrocardiogram	Demonstrates hypertrophy of related cardiac structures	Knowledge deficit: explain all procedures.
Cardiac catheterization	Demonstrates valvular structure and pressures in the heart	Knowledge deficit: explain all procedures

Treatment and Nursing Care

Potential Nursing Diagnoses*

Activity intolerance
Pain (acute)
Ineffective breathing pattern
Risk for infection
Ineffective tissue perfusion (cerebral, peripheral, cardiopulmonary, renal)

BE SMART! Keep patient safe during period of instability by monitoring for syncope, checking for arrhythmias, and preventing falls.

- For the asymptomatic patient, no treatment is required.
- Cardiac glycosides and beta blockers are used to reduce blood volume.
- Surgical repair is the most common treatment when valvular disease becomes symptomatic. Anxiety and fear of the unknown are typical before surgery.
- Cardiac rehabilitation is necessary after valvular replacement. Make sure patient and family understand all medications, physical activity restrictions, nutrition, sexual activity, and prevention of infection.

Appendicitis

Appendicitis is an acute inflammation of the vermiform appendix, a narrow, blind tube that extends from the inferior part of the cecum. The appendix has no known function but does fill and empty as food moves through the gastrointestinal tract. Appendicitis begins when the appendix becomes obstructed or inflamed. Irritation and inflammation lead to engorged veins, stasis, and arterial occlusion. Eventually bacteria accumulate, and the appendix can develop gangrene. Appendicitis is generally caused by obstruction.

Where It Occurs

- The peak incidence of appendicitis occurs between 20 and 30 years of age.
- Twice as many young men as young women develop appendicitis, but after age 25, this ratio gradually diminishes until the gender ratio is even.

Signal Symptoms

- Midabdominal pain (usually right lower quadrant), accompanied by maintaining posture less stressful on the abdomen.
- Abdominal distention.

BE SAFE! If appendicitis is suspected in a female of childbearing age, get a pregnancy test to make sure she does not have an ectopic pregnancy.

Diagnostic Tests

Test	What It Tells	Patient Problems/ Nursing Care
Complete blood count	Infection and inflammation may elevate white blood cell count	Knowledge deficit: explain procedures. Patient will need venipuncture.
Computed tomography of the abdomen with or without contrast	Illustrates enlarged appendix with thickened walls and increased diameter	Knowledge deficit: explain procedures. Patient may need venipuncture or IV line

Treatment and Nursing Care

Potential Nursing Diagnoses*

Pain (acute)

> **BE SMART!** Symptoms of perforation include umbilical pain that moves to the right lower quadrant, nausea, vomiting, loss of appetite, signs of peritonitis (fever, chills, shaking, shock).

- An appendectomy (surgical removal of the appendix) is the preferred method of management for acute appendicitis if the inflammation is localized.
- Crystalloid intravenous fluids are prescribed to replace fluids and electrolytes lost through fever and vomiting.
- Antibiotics control local and systemic infection and reduce the incidence of postoperative wound infection.
- Nursing interventions should focus on promoting patient comfort.

Bowel Obstruction

Bowel obstructions can occur in either the small or large bowel. Small-bowel obstructions (SBOs) have a number of different causes, including postsurgery complications and Crohn's disease. SBOs can be partial or complete and simple or strangulated. Large-bowel obstructions (LBOs) can be caused by interruption of intestinal content flow or colon dilation, the latter leading to a pseudo-obstruction. Cancer and postoperative adhesions are the most common causes of bowel obstruction. Mechanical obstructions are caused by scar tissue (adhesions), twisting or narrowing of the intestines, or hernia.

Where It Occurs

- History of bowel surgery, pelvic surgery, or radiation.
- The incidence of bowel obstructions varies according to the underlying cause.
- SBOs account for 20% of all acute surgical admissions to hospitals.

Signal Symptoms

- LBOs and SBOs usually cause cramping and intermittent pain and significant abdominal distention.
- Colicky pain and vomiting.
- Hyperactive bowel sounds may be present.
- Changes in bowel pattern, diarrhea or constipation.
- Tachycardia, fever.

BE SAFE! If untreated, bowel obstruction can cause bowel strangulation and death.

Diagnostic Tests

Test	What It Tells	Patient Problems/ Nursing Care
Abdominal x-ray	Presence of obstruction; air or fluid in bowel	Knowledge deficit: explain procedures.
Computed tomography scan	Presence of obstruction; air or fluid in bowel	Knowledge deficit: explain procedures.

Treatment and Nursing Care

Potential Nursing Diagnoses*

Pain (acute)
Nausea
Imbalanced nutrition, less than body requirements
Fluid volume deficit

BE SMART! Pain control is important; narcotics such as morphine can be rapidly reversed if needed.

- Antibiotics are used for prophylaxis and analgesics for pain relief.
- Nasogastric tube may be used for severe nausea and vomiting.
- Fluid resuscitation.
- Laparoscopy to relieve obstruction. Surgery may be required depending on location of obstruction.

Cancer, Colorectal

Of cancers of the colon, 65% occur in the rectum and in the sigmoid and descending colon, 25% occur in the cecum and ascending colon, and 10% occur in the transverse colon. Most colorectal tumors (95%) are adenocarcinomas and develop from an adenomatous polyp. Once malignant transformation within the polyp has occurred, the tumor usually grows into the lumen of the bowel, causing obstruction, and invades the deeper layers of the bowel wall. After penetrating the serosa and the mesenteric fat, the tumor may spread by direct extension to nearby organs and the omentum. Metastatic spread through the lymphatic and circulatory systems occurs most frequently to the liver as well as the lung, bones, and brain.

Where It Occurs

- There is a slight predominance of colon cancer in women and rectal cancer in men.
- The incidence increases after age 40 and begins to decline after age 75, although 90% of all newly diagnosed cancers are in people older than 50.

Signal Symptoms

- Rectal bleeding, abdominal pain, changes in bowel patterns.
- Late: bowel sounds may be high pitched, decreased, or absent in the presence of a bowel obstruction.
- Late: distention, ascites, visible masses, or enlarged veins may be present in the abdomen.

BE SAFE! Screening for colon cancer saves lives.

Diagnostic Tests

Test	What It Tells	Patient Problems/ Nursing Care
Hematest	Positive guaiac test for occult blood in the stool is an early sign of tumor development	Knowledge deficit: explain procedures.
Endoscopy of the colon	Visualizes the tumor	Knowledge deficit: explain procedures.

Treatment and Nursing Care

Potential Nursing Diagnoses*

Constipation or diarrhea
Pain (acute)
Risk for infection
Knowledge deficit (medications, surgery, prevention)

BE SMART! A rectal tumor can be easily palpated as the physician performs a digital rectal examination.

■ Surgery is the primary treatment for colorectal cancers.
■ Adjuvant chemotherapy and radiation therapy may be used to improve survival or control symptoms.
■ After surgery, nursing care should focus on providing comfort, preventing complications from major abdominal surgery, and promoting the return of bowel function.
■ Narcotic analgesics manage surgical pain or pain from metastasis.

Cancer, Esophageal

Approximately half of all esophageal cancers are squamous cell carcinomas, which usually occur in the middle and lower two-thirds of the esophagus and are often associated with alcohol and tobacco use. The remaining 50% are adenocarcinomas, which generally begin in glandular tissue of the esophagus. Adenocarcinomas are associated with Barrett's esophagus, a condition that occurs because of continued reflux of fluid from the stomach into the lower esophagus. Over time, reflux changes the cells at the end of the esophagus. Adenocarcinomas may invade the upper portion of the stomach.

Esophageal tumors begin as benign growths and grow rapidly because there is no serosal layer to inhibit growth. Because of the vast lymphatic network of the esophagus, esophageal cancers spread rapidly, both locally to regional lymph nodes and distantly to the lungs and liver. Complications include pulmonary problems that result from fistulae and aspiration; invasion of the tumor into major vessels, causing a massive hemorrhage; and obstruction and compression of the other structures in the head and neck.

Where It Occurs

- Cancer of the esophagus usually occurs between ages 50 and 70 years, and men are affected three times as often as women.
- African Americans are affected three times as often as European Americans, and Asian American men are also at increased risk.

Signal Symptoms

- Dysphagia, weight loss, pain.
- Weakness, persistent cough, hoarseness.

BE SAFE! Make sure that dysphagia and tumor growth do not block the airway or impede breathing.

Diagnostic Tests

Test	What It Tells	Patient Problems/ Nursing Care
Barium swallow	Locates and describes irregularities in the esophageal wall or fistulae	Knowledge deficit: explain procedures. NPO prior to procedures, and expect barium color stools.
Endoscopy	Locates the tumor for a biopsy	Knowledge deficit: explain procedures. NPO prior to procedures, and check for bleeding after the procedure.

Treatment and Nursing Care

Potential Nursing Diagnoses*

Impaired swallowing
Nutrition, imbalanced, less than body requirements
Pain (acute and chronic)
Knowledge deficit (medications, treatment)

> **BE SMART!** Dysphagia is the most common first sign.

- Treatment is often for palliative purposes and to relieve the effects of the tumor.
- Surgery, radiotherapy, and chemotherapy are all options for treating cancer of the esophagus, and they may be used alone or in combination.
- Chemotherapy may be used to kill the cancerous cells.
- Nutritional intake must be monitored and planned.

Cancer, Gallbladder and Pancreatic Duct

Gallbladder cancer and biliary duct cancer are relatively rare and account for fewer than 1% of all cancers. Most cancers of the gallbladder and biliary tract are inoperable at the time of diagnosis. More than 75% of gallbladder cancers are nonpapillary adenocarcinomas, and approximately 6% are papillary adenocarcinomas; a small number are squamous cell, adenosquamous cell, mucinous, or small cell carcinomas.

Biliary system cancer is insidious and metastasizes via the lymphatic and blood systems and by direct extension to the liver, pancreas, stomach, and duodenum. Invasion of the gastrointestinal (GI) tract can cause complete obstruction of the extrahepatic bile ducts with intrahepatic biliary dilation and enlargement of the liver. If the tumor is restricted to one hepatic duct, biliary obstruction is incomplete and jaundice may not be present. Inflammatory disorders such as cholangitis (bile duct inflammation) and peritonitis often obscure an underlying malignancy. Infection often accompanies cancer of the gallbladder, and bile duct cancers are associated with ulcerative colitis.

Where It Occurs

- Biliary system cancer occurs most commonly in individuals in their 70s and occurs two times more frequently in women than in men.
- Gallbladder cancer is more prevalent in Native American and Latin American populations and less so in African Americans.

Signal Symptoms

- Unplanned weight loss, vague GI symptoms.
- Late: thinness, malnourishment, epigastric pain, jaundice from an enlarging tumor that is pressing on the extrahepatic ducts.

BE SAFE! Encourage patient to persist with work-up even when symptoms are vague; often this cancer is diagnosed too late for curative treatment.

Diagnostic Tests

Test	What It Tells	Patient Problems/ Nursing Care
Computed tomography scan	Detects site and size of tumor	Knowledge deficit: explain procedures.
Ultrasonography	Detects site and size of tumor	Knowledge deficit: explain procedures.

Treatment and Nursing Care

Potential Nursing Diagnoses*

Pain (acute and chronic)
Imbalanced nutrition, less than body requirements
Anxiety, death
Disturbed body image

BE SMART! Work with the palliative care service to support patients with disease that requires supportive rather than curative care.

■ Most medical treatment is aimed at supportive care, such as controlling the GI symptoms and the discomforts of jaundice.
■ A cholecystectomy is done as soon as possible after the cancer is detected.
■ Narcotic analgesia is used to control pain.
■ Nursing care should focus on maximizing patient comfort.

Cancer, Liver

Liver cancer, or *hepatocellular carcinoma*, is a malignancy of the liver. Malignant liver tumors (hepatomas) may be classified as primary (arising from the liver parenchyma and almost always associated with an underlying disease of the liver) or secondary (resulting from metastasis from other primary sites). Metastatic disease is far more common than primary liver cancer. Other causes include hepatitis B virus, hepatitis C virus, alcohol, and tobacco.

Chronic liver injury from medications or alcohol misuse may precipitate growth of cancer cells, but the causes of liver cancer are not completely understood.

Where It Occurs

■ Average age of onset is 50 to 60 years.
■ Liver cancer is more common in African and Asian patients.

Signal Symptoms

■ Signs are vague, such as unexplained weight loss and dull, localized ache in the right upper quadrant abdomen; pain may radiate to the right scapula.
■ Late signs: weight loss, ascites, jaundice, liver failure (reduced coagulation, mental status deterioration, general malnutrition, debilitation, risk for infection).

BE SAFE! Intervene aggressively to prevent liver failure from progressing to hepatic encephalopathy (mental status deterioration due to accumulation of metabolic products that cannot be cleared by the liver; lethargy, seizures, tremors, twitching, progressing to coma).

Diagnostic Tests

Test	What It Tells	Patient Problems/ Nursing Care
Liver function tests	Typically demonstrates abnormality	Knowledge deficit: explain procedures. Patient will need venipuncture.
Alpha-fetoprotein	Elevated levels indicate diagnosis	Knowledge deficit: explain procedures. Patient will need venipuncture.

Treatment and Nursing Care

Potential Nursing Diagnoses*

Imbalanced nutrition, less than body requirements
Risk for infection
Impaired tissue integrity
Impaired memory
Pain (acute and chronic)

BE SMART! While primary liver cancer can occur, it is usually a result of metastasis from other sites.

- Surgery (liver resection), radiotherapy, and chemotherapy are all potential treatment methods. The most common therapy is transcatheter arterial chemoembolization (TACE).
- Sedatives and acetaminophen are avoided because poor metabolism can precipitate encephalopathy.
- Esophageal varices (fragile, distended, and thin-walled veins in the esophagus) occur in patients with liver failure because of portal hypertension. Treatment includes surgery and endoscopic sclerotherapy.
- Monitor patient for nutritional deficiencies, bleeding, changes in mental status, skin breakdown, impaired airway, infection.

Cancer, Stomach

Stomach (gastric) cancer is a malignancy that occurs anywhere in the stomach. Infiltration of the lymph nodes, omentum, lungs, and liver may be rapid. Ninety percent of these cancers are adenocarcinomas. Gastric cancer formerly was a leading cause of death worldwide, but those rates have declined with the use of refrigeration. Refrigeration has increased the intake of fruits and vegetables and decreased the intake of processed foods and heavily salted foods. Food preservatives such as nitrates and sulfites may lead to stomach cancer. Refrigeration also decreases bacterial contamination of food. Lower rates of chronic *Helicobacter pylori* infection have also decreased rates of gastric cancer. Smoking is associated with stomach cancer. Five-year survival rate for surgical resection is 30% to 50% for stage II disease and 10% to 25% for stage III disease.

Where It Occurs

- Two-thirds of all cases occur after age 65.
- Incidence of stomach cancer is highest among people from Japan, Iceland, Peru, and Costa Rica.
- Stomach cancer is more common in men than in women.

Signal Symptoms

- Early symptoms: generally vague gastrointestinal symptoms.
- Dysphagia, nausea/vomiting, indigestion.
- Late: postprandial fullness, loss of appetite, melena, hematemesis, obstruction, jaundice, pain, and weight loss.

BE SAFE! Encourage patients to eat a healthy diet; diets with large amounts of processed foods (pickled vegetables, salted fish, and processed meats) are associated with increased risk of gastric cancer.

Diagnostic Tests

Test	What It Tells	Patient Problems/ Nursing Care
Hematology	Anemias are common in ulcerated lesions; eosinophilia and polycythemia may be seen	Knowledge deficit: explain procedures. Patient will need venipuncture.
Chemistry with liver function	Rules out liver involvement	Knowledge deficit: explain procedures. Patient will need venipuncture.

Treatment and Nursing Care

Potential Nursing Diagnoses*

Nausea

Constipation

Diarrhea

Knowledge deficit (pre- and postoperative education, treatment options, nutrition, smoking cessation)

BE SMART! Provide pre- and postoperative teaching for all patients undergoing gastric surgery.

- Surgery is commonly done: depending on site, the following surgeries are common: total gastrectomy, esophagogastrectomy for tumors of the cardia and gastroesophageal junction, and a subtotal gastrectomy for cancers of the distal stomach.
- Chemotherapy and radiation therapy have little effect.
- Smoking cessation is important.

Colitis

Ulcerative colitis is a chronic inflammatory disease of the colon. Usually, the disease begins in the rectum and sigmoid colon and gradually spreads up the colon in a continuous distribution pattern. The inflammatory process involves the mucosa and submucosa of the colon, and causes are mostly speculative in nature but include infection, hypersensitivity to various allergens, ischemia, vasculitis, or drugs.

Gradually, multiple ulcerations and abscesses form at the inflamed areas. As the disease progresses, the colon mucosa becomes edematous and thickened with scar tissue formation, which results in altered absorptive capabilities of the colon. The severity of the disease ranges from a mild form that is localized in specific areas of the bowel to a critical syndrome with life-threatening complications. The most common complications are nutritional deficiencies; others include sepsis, fistulae, abscesses, and hemorrhage. For unknown reasons, patients with ulcerative colitis also have a high risk for arthritis and cancer.

Where It Occurs

- The peak incidence occurs during the early adolescent and young adult years, often between ages 10 and 15 years.
- Girls are infected more often than boys.
- Evidence suggests a second peak incidence among those 55 to 60 years of age.
- Asian Americans appear to have lower incidence rates.

Signal Symptoms

- Abdominal pain, tenderness, distention, guarding.
- Blood and mucus in the stool.
- Fever, chills.
- Late: signs of malnutrition and dehydration (dry mucous membranes, poor skin turgor, muscle weakness, and lethargy).

BE SAFE! Infections should be treated promptly so that they do not progress to more serious conditions such as peritonitis and sepsis.

Diagnostic Tests

Test	What It Tells	Patient Problems/ Nursing Care
Colonoscopy; sigmoidoscopy	Direct visualization of mucosa by endoscopic examination	Knowledge deficit: explain procedures, including gastrointestinal prepping and NPO.
Barium enema with air contrast	Fluoroscopic and radiographic examination of large intestine after rectal instillation of barium sulfate to identify structural abnormalities (use with caution in severe cases)	Knowledge deficit: explain procedures, including gastrointestinal prepping and NPO.

Treatment and Nursing Care

Potential Nursing Diagnoses*

Alteration in nutrition
Risk for infection
Pain (acute)
Diarrhea

BE SMART! Provide a nutritional consultation to make sure the patient understands dietary modifications.

- Mesalamine and similar medications are used as anti-inflammatory agents. Antibiotics are used to treat infection.
- In acute situations, stop feedings, initiate nasogastric decompression, and begin intravenous fluid resuscitation along with electrolytes replacement and acid-base balance.
- Surgery may be performed when patients fail to respond to conservative treatment.
- Nursing care focuses on promoting physical and emotional comfort for the patient.

Colostomy and Ileostomy

Colostomies and ileostomies are surgical stomas that connect a body cavity to the skin's surface and are named according to their anatomical location. Thus, a *colostomy* is a surgical procedure whereby the surgeon creates a stoma by attaching a loop of the large intestine, the colon, to the surface of the skin. The *ileostomy* is a surgical procedure whereby a loop of the small intestine, or ileum, is brought to the surface of the skin. These procedures are performed when disease or injury makes portions of the gastrointestinal tract incapable of processing intestinal waste.

Where It Occurs

- Diseases of the large intestine that might require ileostomy include ulcerative colitis, colorectal cancer, and Crohn's disease.
- Diseases of the large intestine that might require colostomy include colorectal cancer and diverticulitis.

Signal Symptoms

- Potential complications: infection, leakage of intestinal contents, fecal odor, bleeding, hernia at site of stoma, scar tissue, skin breakdown.

BE SAFE! Observe new stomas for signs of poor perfusion (pallor), bleeding, and infection.

Diagnostic Tests

Test	What It Tells	Patient Problems/ Nursing Care
Colonoscopy or a sigmoidoscopy	To identify anatomy and perform laparoscopic-assisted loop colostomy	Knowledge deficit: explain procedures. Complete pre-operative preparation. NPO.

Treatment and Nursing Care

Potential Nursing Diagnoses*

Risk for constipation
Risk for infection
Disturbed body image
Knowledge deficit (colostomy management, nutrition and diet,
  medications)

BE SMART! The patient experiences altered body image and
needs to learn strategies to maintain quality of life.

- Surgical location is critical because poor location of the stoma
  can lead to poor self-management. Pre-operative marking of the
  stoma site is important for placement of the ostomy appliance with
  adequate seal and drainage. The stoma should be placed away from
  the umbilicus, skin folds in obese patients, and bony prominences.
- Teach patient to manage ostomy care, eat a well-balanced diet,
  monitor medications, manage drainage, and complete irrigation
  if appropriate.

Crohn's Disease

Crohn's disease (CD), also known as *granulomatous colitis* or *regional
enteritis*, is a chronic, nonspecific inflammatory disease of the bowel
that occurs most commonly in the terminal ileum, jejunum, and colon,
although it may affect any part of the gastrointestinal (GI) system from
the mouth to the anus. Like ulcerative colitis, CD is marked by remissions
and exacerbations, but, unlike ulcerative colitis, it can affect any portion
of the tubular GI tract. Research has not established a specific cause for
CD, but the following situations may contribute: genetic predisposition,
environmental factors, diet, immune factors, smoking, oral conceptive
use, and use of NSAIDs.

The disease creates deep, longitudinal mucosal ulcerations and nodular submucosal thickenings called *granulomas*, which give the intestinal
wall a cobblestone appearance and may alter its absorptive abilities. The
inflamed and ulcerated areas occur only in segments of the bowel, and

normal bowel tissue segments occur between the diseased segments. Eventually, thickening of the bowel wall, narrowing of the bowel lumen, and strictures of the bowel are common. Also, fistulae that connect to other tissue—such as the skin, bladder, rectum, and vagina—often occur.

Where It Occurs

- Rates are slightly higher in males.
- CD is more common in whites than in African Americans or Asian Americans.
- There is a twofold to fourfold increase in the prevalence of CD in the Jewish population in the United States and Europe as compared with other groups.

Signal Symptoms

- Fever, prolonged diarrhea containing blood and pus, abdominal pain (right lower quadrant), weight loss, fatigue.
- Malnutrition and dehydration.

BE SAFE! Assess for signs of intestinal obstruction due to bowel inflammation and edema: cramping, bloating, pain, loud bowel sounds.

Diagnostic Tests

Test	What It Tells	Patient Problems/ Nursing Care
Upper GI and barium enema series	Determines the location and extent of rectal involvement, including inflammation strictures, perianal disease, and fistulae	Knowledge deficit: explain procedures, including gastrointestinal prepping and NPO.
Sigmoidoscopy or colonoscopy	Detects location of illness, early mucosal changes, inflammation, strictures, and fistulae	Knowledge deficit: explain procedures, including gastrointestinal prepping and NPO.

Treatment and Nursing Care

Potential Nursing Diagnoses*

Imbalanced nutrition, less than body requirements
Diarrhea
Disturbed body image
Anxiety

BE SMART! Encourage compliance with colonoscopy recommendations; risk of adenocarcinoma of the colon in Crohn's colitis is 4 to 20 times that for the general population.

- Mesalamine is commonly prescribed as an anti-inflammatory agent. Other anti-inflammatory agents, antibiotics, and antidiarrheal agents are often needed.
- Most patients have surgical procedures at some point to remove inflamed portions of the bowel. Conservation of functional bowel is a high priority. Surgery may be needed for intestinal obstruction, perforation, abscesses, or fistulae.
- During acute exacerbations, bowel rest is important to promote healing.
- Balanced diet with overnight feeding is used for patients with reduced appetite.
- Nursing care focuses on supporting the patient through acute episodes of inflammation and teaching measures to prevent future inflammatory attacks.

Diverticular Disease

Diverticular disease has two clinical forms: *diverticulosis* and *diverticulitis*. People with diverticulosis have multiple, noninflamed diverticula (outpouches of the intestinal mucosa through the circular smooth muscle of the bowel wall). Usually, diverticulosis is asymptomatic and does not require treatment. Diverticulitis, in contrast, occurs when the diverticula become inflamed or microperforated. Diverticular disease usually occurs in the descending and sigmoid colons and is accompanied by signs of inflammation.

Patients generally have increased muscular contractions in the sigmoid colon that produce muscular thickness and increased intraluminal pressure. This increased pressure, accompanied by a weakness in the colon wall, causes diverticular formations.

Where It Occurs

- From 30% to 60% of people with diverticular disease are between 60 and 80 years old. Incidence increases with age.
- Diverticular disease is rare in those under age 40.
- Prevalence is the same for men and women.
- Although its cause is uncertain, diverticular disease is associated with low-fiber diet, constipation, and obesity.

Signal Symptoms

- Crampy pain, changes in bowel habits, nausea and vomiting, constipation, diarrhea, flatulence, and bloating.
- Malnutrition: weight loss, lethargy, brittle nails, and hair loss.
- Temperature and pulse elevations.

BE SAFE! Signs of ruptured diverticuli and peritonitis include pain, fever, chills, abdominal distention and guarding, diarrhea; these signs should be acted on promptly.

Diagnostic Tests

Test	What It Tells	Patient Problems/ Nursing Care
Computed tomography (test of choice) and magnetic resonance imaging	Locates abnormalities such as diverticula, abscesses, fistulas, and pericolic fat inflammation	Knowledge deficit: explain procedures.
Technetium-99m sodium pertechnetate (gastric or Meckel's) scan	Highlights the presence of mucosal abnormalities and may demonstrate diverticula	Knowledge deficit: explain procedures; venipuncture may be required.

Potential Nursing Diagnoses*

Pain (acute)
Anxiety
Nausea
Diarrhea
Knowledge deficit (medications, nutrition)

BE SMART! Palpate for a mass in the lower left quadrant of the abdomen, which may indicate diverticular inflammation.

- For uncomplicated diverticulosis, a diet high in vegetable fiber is recommended.
- Surgical intervention may be required if the diverticular disease becomes symptomatic and is not relieved with conservative treatment.
- Anticholinergic drugs control pain by diminishing colon spasms.
- Oral antibiotics control the spread of infection when a fever is present.
- For uncomplicated diverticulosis, nursing interventions focus on teaching measures to prevent acute inflammatory episodes.

Esophageal Varices

Esophageal varices are abnormally dilated veins of the esophagus. Esophageal varices may be uphill or downhill depending on blood flow. Uphill varices, which are more prevalent, are caused by portal hypertension. Downhill varices are caused by superior vena cava blockage.

Approximately 1,500 mL/min of blood is transported by the portal vein from the GI tract to the liver and, with obstruction in a diseased liver, causes an increase in portal venous pressure and development of a collateral circulation. Normal portal pressure ranges from 5 and 10 mm Hg, and once it increases above 12 mm Hg, varices and ascites can occur. As esophageal varices expand, they can rupture and bleed profusely.

Where It Occurs

■ Esophageal varices are generally found with liver failure, hepatitis B and C, and cirrhosis. Cirrhosis is the most common cause.
■ Patients with excessive alcohol use are at risk for liver failure, portal hypertension, and esophageal varices.

Signal Symptoms

■ Liver failure: fatigue, anorexia, nausea, vomiting, weight loss, abdominal discomfort, jaundice, edema, pruritus.
■ Spontaneous bleeding, easy bruising, retching, bloody vomiting, hematemesis, and melena.
■ Signs of shock: pallor, tachycardia, postural hypotension, delayed capillary refill, cool extremities, shortness of breath, deteriorating mental status.

BE SAFE! Monitor the amount and type of bleeding; obtain intravenous access to provide fluid resuscitation.

Diagnostic Tests

Test	What It Tells	Patient Problems/ Nursing Care
Endoscopy	Visualizes esophageal varices	Knowledge deficit: explain procedures. Sedation is needed. NPO.
Liver function tests, complete blood count	Determines liver function and amount of blood loss	Knowledge deficit: explain procedures. Patient will need venipuncture.

Treatment and Nursing Care

Potential Nursing Diagnoses*

Fluid volume deficit
Ineffective airway clearance
Risk for aspiration

Ineffective breathing pattern
Anxiety

BE SMART! Take the blood pressure and pulse when the patient is lying and sitting to determine if postural hypotension exists.

- If patients have no previous history of esophageal varices, they may receive nonselective beta-adrenergic blockers.
- Endoscopic sclerotherapy or variceal ligation is successful to treat variceal bleeding.
- Provide intravenous fluids and blood products to support the circulation.
- Type and crossmatch the patient for possible blood and platelet transfusions. Keep blood on standby in case of emergency.
- Consider airway protection with an endotracheal tube in case of vomiting.
- Balloon tamponade and surgery might be necessary for continued bleeding.
- Nursing care focuses on protection of the airway and fluid resuscitation during the acute phase and patient teaching as the patient recovers.

Esophagitis

Esophagitis is inflammation of the lining of the esophagus that leads to swelling and pain and, ultimately, scarring. It is caused by bacteria, fungi, viruses, or chronic reflex of stomach contents. Esophagitis is most commonly the result of gastroesophageal reflux disease (GERD).

Where It Occurs

- Esophagitis is usually observed in adults, not children.
- Pregnancy; obesity; cigarette smoking; alcohol misuse and abuse; ingestion of chocolate, high fat, and spicy foods; scleroderma.
- Medications: beta blocker, NSAIDs, caffeine, theophylline.
- Infectious agents, especially viruses and candida.

Signal Symptoms

- Heartburn that gets worse with tight clothing and a reflux of gastric contents.
- Abdominal discomfort, difficulty swallowing, cough, hoarseness, wheezing, nausea, bloating, and fullness.
- Midsternal pain radiating to the arm that is similar to cardiac chest pain.

BE SAFE! Pain from esophagitis mimics cardiac chest pain, at times complicating assessment.

Diagnostic Tests

Test	What It Tells	Patient Problems/ Nursing Care
Endoscopy	Direct visualization of mucosa by endoscopic examination	Knowledge deficit: explain procedures, including gastrointestinal prepping before test. NPO.

Treatment and Nursing Care

Potential Nursing Diagnoses*

Pain (acute)
Nausea
Risk for infection
Impaired oral mucous membrane
Imbalanced nutrition, less than body requirements

BE SMART! Teaching about the type and dose of medications is an important strategy.

- Treatment varies according to the underlying cause and is often medicinal. Proton pump inhibitors are usually used.
- If esophagitis is fungal in origin, antifungal agents are used.
- Pain relief is important.
- Teach patients about strategies for pain relief and the rationale and dosage of all medications.

Gall Bladder Disease: Cholecystitis and Cholelithiasis

Cholecystitis is an inflammation of the gallbladder wall; it may be either acute or chronic. It is almost always associated with cholelithiasis, or gallstones, which lodge in the gallbladder, cystic duct, or common bile duct. Silent gallstones are so common that most of the American public may have them at some time; only stones that are symptomatic require treatment.

Gallstones are most commonly made of either cholesterol or bilirubin and calcium. If gallstones obstruct the neck of the gallbladder or the cystic duct, the gallbladder can become infected with bacteria such as *Escherichia coli*. The primary agents, however, are not the bacteria but mediators such as members of the prostaglandin family. The gallbladder becomes enlarged up to two to three times normal, causing decreased tissue perfusion. If the gallbladder becomes ischemic as well as infected, necrosis, perforation, and sepsis can follow.

Where It Occurs

- The incidence of gallbladder disease increases with age; most patients are middle-aged or older women.
- Northern European, Native American, or Hispanic/Latino ancestry are all risk factors.
- Children with sickle cell disease or on total parenteral nutrition are at risk.

Signal Symptoms

- Severe upper abdominal pain, colicky pain.
- Jaundice, low-grade fever.
- Positive Murphy's sign (positive palpation of a distended gallbladder during inhalation).

BE SAFE! Acute attacks are often followed by residual aching or soreness for up to 24 hours.

Diagnostic Tests

Test	What It Tells	Patient Problems/ Nursing Care
White blood cell (WBC) count	Infection and inflammation elevate the WBC count	Knowledge deficit: explain procedures. Patient will need venipuncture.
Ultrasound scan	Illustrates gallbladder wall thickening, presence of gallstones, and pericholecystic fluid collections	Knowledge deficit: explain procedures.

Treatment and Nursing Care

Potential Nursing Diagnoses*

Pain (acute)
Risk for infection
Anxiety
Fluid volume deficit

> **BE SMART!** Elderly patients, especially those with diabetes, may have vague symptoms such as low-grade fever and localized tenderness. In the elderly, the condition may progress rapidly to sepsis.

- Medical management may include oral bile acid therapy.
- There are several surgical or procedural treatment options, such as a laparoscopic cholecystectomy.
- Antibiotics may be prescribed to manage bacteria that are typical bowel flora.
- If surgery is required, the nurse's first priority is the maintenance of airway, breathing, and circulation.

Gastritis

Gastritis is any inflammatory process of the mucosal lining of the stomach. The inflammation may be contained within one region or be patchy in many areas. Gastric structure and function are altered in either the epithelial or the glandular components of the gastric mucosa. The inflammation is usually limited to the mucosa, but some forms involve the deeper layers of the gastric wall. Gastritis is classified into acute, most commonly caused by alcohol abuse or ingestion of NSAIDs, and chronic, typically considered an autoimmune disorder.

The most common form of acute gastritis is acute hemorrhagic gastritis, also called *acute erosive gastritis*. The gastric erosions are limited to the mucosa, which have edema and sites of bleeding. Erosions can be diffuse throughout the stomach or localized to the antrum. The three forms of chronic inflammation of the gastric mucosa are *superficial gastritis*, *atrophic gastritis*, and *gastric atrophy*. Chronic gastritis has also been classified as type A and type B. Type A chronic gastritis, the less common form, involves the body of the stomach (fundus) rather than the antrum. Type B gastritis is a more common nonautoimmune inflammation of the lining of the stomach. It primarily involves the antrum but can affect the entire stomach as age increases.

Where It Occurs

- Acute: occurs in men more than in women; is caused by *Helicobacter pylori* infection and autoimmune deficiency in cobalamin.
- Chronic: occurs more frequently in women than in men; is caused by *H. pylori* infection, allergies, alcohol; bacterial, viral, and fungal infections; and acute stress with shock.
- The incidence is highest in the ages between 50 and 70.
- Men and women who are heavy smokers and alcohol abusers are at particular risk.
- Autoimmune gastritis occurs more often in people of northern European descent and with African American ancestry and is less frequent in southern Europeans and Asians.

Signal Symptoms

- Nausea, vomiting, sensation of fullness, epigastric pain, flatulence.
- Fever, dehydration, thirst.
- Upper GI bleeding, pallor.
- Tachycardia, hypotension, hematemesis, and melena.

BE SAFE! The condition can be aggravated by or caused by the use of NSAIDs, which irritate the stomach mucosal.

Diagnostic Tests

Test	What It Tells	Patient Problems/ Nursing Care
Esophagogastroduodenoscopy with biopsy	Visualization of inflamed gastric mucosa; biopsy results show the specific type of gastritis	Knowledge deficit: explain procedures, including NPO. Observe for bleeding.

Treatment and Nursing Care

Potential Nursing Diagnoses*

Imbalanced nutrition, less than body requirements
Pain (acute)
Fluid volume deficit
Risk for infection

BE SMART! Teach patients to take prescribed medications and avoid drugs that can worsen inflammation.

- The immediate treatment for acute gastritis is directed toward alleviating the symptoms and withdrawing the causative agents.
- If hemorrhaging is profuse and persistent, blood replacement is necessary.
- For *H. pylori* infections, two antibiotics, such as clarithromycin (Biaxin), amoxicillin, tetracycline, or metronidazole (Flagyl), are usually prescribed.
- Proton pump inhibitors, such as omeprazole (Prilosec), lansoprazole (Prevacid), or esomeprazole (Nexium) are usually prescribed; H_2 receptor antagonist may be used to block gastric secretion and maintain the pH of gastric contents above 4.0, thereby decreasing inflammation.

- Sulcrafate (Carafate) forms an adhesive gel to protect damaged gastric mucosa.
- Nurses should educate patients about what food and substances to avoid consuming.

Gastroesophageal Reflux Disease

Gastroesophageal reflux disease (GERD) is a syndrome caused by esophageal reflux, or the backward flow of gastroesophageal contents into the esophagus. GERD occurs because of inappropriate relaxation of the lower esophageal sphincter (LES) in response to an unknown stimulus. Reflux occurs in most adults, but if it occurs regularly, the esophagus cannot resist the irritating effects of gastric acid and pepsin because the mucosal barrier of the esophagus breaks down. Without this protection, tissue injury, inflammation, hyperemia, and even erosion occur.

As healing occurs, the cells that replace the normal squamous cell epithelium may be more resistant to reflux but may also be a premalignant tissue that can lead to adenocarcinoma. Repeated exposure may also lead to fibrosis and scarring, which can cause esophageal stricture to occur. Stricture leads to difficulty in swallowing. Chronic reflux is often associated with hiatus hernia. Barrett's esophagus is a condition thought to be caused by the chronic reflux of gastric acid into the esophagus. It occurs when squamous epithelium of the esophagus is replaced by intestinal columnar epithelium, a situation that may lead to adenocarcinoma. Barrett's esophagus is present in approximately 10% to 15% of patients with GERD.

Where It Occurs

- GERD occurs at any age but is most common in people over 50.
- Although white males are more at risk than other populations for Barrett's esophagus and adenocarcinoma, no gender or racial/ethnic considerations are reported for other types of gastroesophageal reflux.

Signal Symptoms

- Heartburn, regurgitation, and difficulty swallowing.
- Noncardiac chest pain, cough, clearing of throat, hoarseness, and aspiration.
- Asthma, pneumonia.

BE SAFE! Pain from GERD mimics cardiac chest pain, at times complicating assessment.

Diagnostic Tests

Test	What It Tells	Patient Problems/ Nursing Care
Esophageal pH monitoring	Presence of gastric contents in the esophagus decreases pH	Knowledge deficit: explain procedures.
Esophageal manometry	Multilumen esophageal catheter introduced through mouth and used to measure esophageal pressures during a variety of swallowing maneuvers	Knowledge deficit: explain procedures, including gastrointestinal prepping and NPO.

Treatment and Nursing Care

Potential Nursing Diagnoses*

Pain (acute)
Nausea
Risk for infection
Impaired oral mucous membrane
Imbalanced nutrition, less than body requirements

BE SMART! Teaching about the type and dose of medications is an important strategy.

- Although diet therapy alone can manage symptoms in some patients, most patients can have their GERD managed pharmacologically.
- Antacids neutralize gastric acid and relieve heartburn.

■ Proton pump inhibitors (thought to be more effective than antacids), or H_2 receptor antagonists, block the final step in the H^+ ion secretion by the parietal cell; they have few adverse effects and are well tolerated.

Gastrointestinal Hemorrhage

Gastrointestinal hemorrhaging can be classified as either upper or lower, depending on the location of the bleeding. Upper GI bleed (UGIB) is bleeding of recent origin that occurs before the ligament of Treitz; lower GI bleed (LGIB) occurs beyond the ligament of Treitz.

UGIB can be caused by dyspepsia (especially nocturnal symptoms), ulcer disease, alcohol misuse and abuse, anticoagulation, and NSAID or aspirin use. In these conditions, tears in the upper GI tract occur or varices become distended and bleed. LGIB occurs from diverticulosis, hemorrhoids, tumors, liver disease, ischemic colitis, anticoagulation, and NSAID use. In these conditions, a blood vessel becomes perforated, lacerated, or damaged by the disease process.

Where It Occurs

■ UGIB and LGIB are found in twice as many men as women in the United States and United Kingdom.
■ Both are more common in the elderly.

Signal Symptoms

■ UGIB: vomiting blood or hematemesis (coffee ground emesis), black stools with foul odor, melena. Other symptoms include dyspepsia, sensation of fullness.
■ LGIB: bloody (red wine–colored) stool.
■ Syncope, dizziness, tachycardia, hypotension, diaphoresis, delayed capillary refill, decreased urine output.

BE SAFE! The primary risk is an arterial hemorrhage, which needs to be treated rapidly.

Diagnostic Tests

Test	What It Tells	Patient Problems/ Nursing Care
Colonoscopy	Presence of bleeding in lower gastrointestinal regions	Knowledge deficit: explain procedures, including gastrointestinal prepping and NPO.
Endoscopy	Presence of bleeding in upper gastrointestinal regions	Knowledge deficit: explain procedures, including gastrointestinal prepping and NPO.

Treatment and Nursing Care

Potential Nursing Diagnoses*

Fluid volume deficit
Ineffective airway clearance
Risk for aspiration
Ineffective breathing pattern
Anxiety

BE SMART! Maintenance of airway and fluid volume resuscitation are the highest priorities in a UGIB.

- UGIB: Decompression of the upper GI with a nasogastric tube; surgery may be performed to oversew the bleeding vessel, or embolization may be used. Cyclooxygenase-2 inhibitors; irradication of *Helicobacter pylori with antibiotics.*
- Vasopressin infusion may stop bleeding through vasoconstriction.
- Orthostatic hypotension (blood pressure fall of >10 mm Hg when patient goes from lying to sitting position) generally shows blood loss of more than 1,000 mL in both UGIB and LGIB.
- LGIB is generally treated with surgery if bleeding progresses. Embolization with substances such as gelatin sponge or polyvinyl alcohol may be used.
- Nursing care focuses on maintaining patent airway, providing fluid and blood resuscitation, and teaching patient to prevent recurrences.

Hepatic Cirrhosis

Cirrhosis is a chronic liver disease characterized by destruction of the functional liver cells, which leads to cellular death. Liver cirrhosis is most commonly associated with hepatitis C (26% of the cases), alcohol abuse (21%), hepatitis C plus alcohol abuse (15%), cryptogenic causes (etiology not determined; 18%), hepatitis B (15%), and other miscellaneous causes (5%). In cirrhosis, the damaged liver cells regenerate as fibrotic areas instead of functional cells, causing lymph damage and alterations in liver structure, function, and blood circulation. The major cellular changes include irreversible chronic injury of the functional liver tissue and the formation of regenerative nodules. These changes result in liver cell necrosis, collapse of liver support networks, distortion of the vascular bed, and nodular regeneration of the remaining liver cells.

The classification of cirrhosis is controversial, but most types may be classified by a mixture of causes and cellular changes, defined as follows: alcoholic; cryptogenic and postviral or postnecrotic; biliary; cardiac; metabolic, inherited, and drug related; and miscellaneous.

Where It Occurs

- Cirrhosis is most commonly seen in the middle-aged population and is more common in males than in females.
- Hepatitis C is more prevalent in minority populations, such as African Americans and Hispanic persons, than in other populations.
- Alcohol dependence and alcoholic liver disease are more common in minority groups, particularly among Native Americans.

Signal Symptoms

- Ascites, weight loss, nausea, vomiting, fatigue, pruritus, right upper quadrant pain.
- Poor skin turgor, signs of jaundice, bruising, spider angiomas, and palmar erythema (reddened palms).
- Asterixis (liver flap or flapping tremor), decreased mental status progressing to coma.

BE SAFE! Increasing liver failure can progress quickly and lead to decreased mental status and coma. Monitor neurological status carefully.

Diagnostic Tests

Test	What It Tells	Patient Problems/ Nursing Care
Percutaneous or laparoscopic liver needle biopsy	Distinguishes advanced liver disease from cirrhosis	Knowledge deficit: explain procedures. Observe for bleeding and infection and medicate for pain.
Liver enzymes: aspartate aminotransferase (AST); alanine aminotransferase (ALT); lactate dehydrogenase (LDH)	Liver cellular dysfunction leads to accumulation of enzymes	Knowledge deficit: explain procedures. Patient will need venipuncture.

Treatment and Nursing Care

Potential Nursing Diagnoses*

Fluid volume excess
Pain (acute)
Activity intolerance
Impaired skin integrity
Imbalanced nutrition, less than body requirements
Risk for infection

BE SMART! Assess patients for alcohol withdrawal; if signs of increased irritability and restlessness occur, consider preventing delirium tremens with benzodiazepines.

- Patients are placed on a well-balanced, high-calorie, moderate- to high-protein, low-fat, low-sodium diet with additional vitamins and folic acid.
- Surgical intervention includes a LeVeen continuous peritoneal jugular shunt (peritoneovenous shunt) and, in some cases, liver transplantation.

- Nursing considerations in the cirrhotic patient are to avoid infection and circulatory problems.
- Patient teaching includes nutrition, physical activity, skin care, eliminating alcohol use.

Hepatic Failure

Liver (hepatic) failure is a loss of liver function because of the death of many hepatocytes. The damage can occur suddenly, as with a viral infection, or slowly over time, as with cirrhosis. Acute liver failure refers to both fulminant hepatic failure (FHF) and subfulminant hepatic failure. FHF occurs when sudden (within 8 weeks from onset), severe liver decompensation caused by massive necrosis of the liver leads to coagulopathies and encephalopathy. Subfulminant hepatic failure, also known as *late-onset hepatic failure*, is considered late onset because it can take up to 26 weeks before hepatic encephalopathy develops. Hepatic encephalopathy occurs with neurological changes such as personality changes, changes in cognition and intellect, and reduced level of consciousness.

Because of the complex functions of the liver, liver failure leads to multiple system complications. When ammonia and other metabolic by-products are not metabolized, they accumulate in the blood and cause neurological deterioration. Without normal vitamin K activation and the production of clotting factors, the patient has coagulation problems. Patients are at risk for infections because of general malnutrition, debilitation, impairment of phagocytosis, and decreased liver production of immune-related proteins. Fluid retention occurs because of decreased albumin production, leading to decreased colloidal osmotic pressure with failure to retain fluid in the bloodstream. Renin and aldosterone production cause sodium and water retention. Ascites occurs because of intrahepatic vascular obstruction with fluid movement into the peritoneum.

Where It Occurs

- Infants and children are more likely to have an inherited disease, whereas adult men are more likely to have alcohol-related disease.
- Worldwide statistics indicate that postnecrotic cirrhosis is more common in women than in men.

Signal Symptoms

- Ascites, weight loss, nausea, vomiting, fatigue, pruritus, right upper quadrant pain.
- Poor skin turgor, signs of jaundice, bruising, spider angiomas, and palmar erythema (reddened palms).
- Asterixis (liver flap or flapping tremor), decreased mental status progressing to coma.

BE SAFE! Increasing liver failure can progress quickly and lead to decreased mental status and coma. Monitor neurological status carefully.

Diagnostic Tests

Test	What It Tells	Patient Problems/ Nursing Care
Prothrombin time	Prolonged time indicates liver dysfunction	Knowledge deficit: explain procedures. Patient will need venipuncture.
Viral hepatitis serologies	Identify patients with hepatitis	Knowledge deficit: explain procedures. Patient will need venipuncture.

Treatment and Nursing Care

Potential Nursing Diagnoses*

Fluid volume excess
Pain (acute)
Activity intolerance
Impaired skin integrity
Imbalanced nutrition, less than body requirements
Risk for infection

BE SMART! Refer the patient to palliative care and pay particular attention to nutrition and adequate rest for the patient.

- Liver transplantation is the definitive treatment for liver failure.
- Histamine (H_2) receptor antagonists decrease gastric secretion and are used as prophylaxis for ulcers.
- Patients are placed on a well-balanced, high-calorie, moderate-to high-protein, low-fat, low-sodium diet with additional vitamins and folic acid.
- Patient teaching includes nutrition, physical activity, skin care, eliminating alcohol use.
- Thiamine reduces risk for neuropathies.
- Nursing care focuses on monitoring fluid volume excess and airway compromise.

Hepatitis

Hepatitis is a widespread inflammation of the liver that results in degeneration and necrosis of liver cells. In general, the majority of cases of hepatitis are self-limiting and resolve without complications. Hospitalization is required only when symptoms are severe, persistent, or debilitating. Approximately 20% of acute hepatitis B and 50% of hepatitis C cases progress to a chronic state. The most serious complication of hepatitis is fulminant hepatitis, which occurs in approximately 1% of all patients and leads to liver failure and hepatic encephalopathy and, in some, to death within 2 weeks of onset. Other complications include a syndrome that resembles serum sickness (muscle and joint pain, rash, angioedema), as well as cirrhosis, pancreatitis, myocarditis, aplastic anemia, or peripheral neuropathy.

Hepatitis can be caused by bacteria, by hepatotoxic agents (drugs, alcohol, industrial chemicals), or most commonly, by a virus. Infection with both hepatitis B virus and HIV is common. Up to 90% of HIV-infected individuals either have had a previous hepatitis B infection or have a current, active one.

Where It Occurs

- Children 5 to 14 years of age are most likely to acquire acute hepatitis A virus (HAV) infection.
- Hepatitis B virus (HBV) and hepatitis C virus (HCV) have higher prevalence among African Americans and persons of Hispanic/Latino origin than among other populations.
- Hepatitis D virus (HDV) infection is more common in adults than in children.

Signal Symptoms

- Flu-like symptoms, fever (generally 101°F to 102°F), malaise, weakness, fatigue.
- Enlarged and tender liver, jaundice, anorexia, nausea, vomiting, bleeding tendencies.
- Dark urine, pale stool.

BE SAFE! At-risk populations such as men who have sex with men who test positive for HAV and HBV should also be tested for HIV given the association of the diseases.

Diagnostic Tests

Test	What It Tells	Patient Problems/ Nursing Care
Viral hepatitis serologies	Identify immune response to virus leads to markers such as immunoglobulins (IgG and IgM), antigens, antibodies	Knowledge deficit: explain procedures. Patient will need venipuncture.
Liver function tests	Determine the extent of inflammation	Knowledge deficit: explain procedures. Patient will need venipuncture.

Treatment and Nursing Care

Potential Nursing Diagnoses*

Impaired skin integrity
Imbalanced nutrition, less than body requirements
Risk for infection
Pain (acute)
Activity intolerance

BE SMART! Health-care providers who are exposed to blood and body fluids should receive the hepatitis vaccine (hepatitis A and B).

- Hepatitis A is generally treated supportively by treating symptoms such as nausea, fatigue, and dehydration.
- Hepatitis B may be treated with antivirals or interferons.
- Antivirals for HBV and HCV reduce viral replication.
- Interferons: alpha, beta, and gamma for HBV and HCV bind with receptors to modulate host-immune response.
- Nurses focus on providing education about prevention, medications, pain relief and comfort.

Hernia

A hernia, often called a *rupture*, is a protrusion or projection of an organ or organ part through the wall of the cavity that normally contains it. Hernias tend to be caused by congenital or acquired weakness of the abdomen wall. Types of hernias include direct or indirect, ventral or incisional, hiatal, traumatic, irreducible or incarcerated (contents cannot be replaced into the abdomen), and strangulated (irreducible hernia in which the blood supply to the entrapped bowel loop is compromised). Hernias are also classified according to location, such as inguinal, femoral, or umbilical. An inguinal hernia occurs when either the omentum, the large or small intestine, or the bladder protrudes into the inguinal canal.

Where It Occurs

- Umbilical and femoral hernias occur more frequently in women.
- Indirect inguinal hernias are 8 to 10 times more common in men.
- Hernias occur in both children and adults. Low-birth-weight and male infants are at higher risk for this defect than are female infants or full-term infants.

Signal Symptoms

- Bulge along the inguinal area, which is especially apparent when the patient coughs or strains. The swelling may subside on its own when the patient assumes a recumbent position or if slight manual pressure is applied externally to the area.
- Steady aching pain.

BE SAFE! Absent bowel sounds suggests strangulation of the hernia

Diagnostic Tests

Test	What It Tells	Patient Problems/ Nursing Care
Abdominal ultrasonography	Location of outpouching	Knowledge deficit: explain procedure.

Treatment and Nursing Care

Potential Nursing Diagnoses*

Ineffective tissue perfusion (abdominal)
Risk for infection
Pain (acute and chronic)
Knowledge deficit (postoperative management)

BE SMART! Usually the diagnosis is made by physical examination.

- Surgical hernia repair is often recommended. Following surgery, provide pain management and surveillance for infection.
- Abdominal truss may be used as an alternative treatment method.
- If no surgery is done, teach the signs of a strangulated or incarcerated hernia: severe pain, nausea, vomiting, diarrhea, high fever, and bloody stools. Explain that if these symptoms occur, the patient must notify the primary health-care provider immediately.

Inflammatory Bowel Disease

Inflammatory bowel disease (IBD) is a general term for a chronic, episodic, inflammatory disorder of various portions of the bowel. IBD is divided into two major categories: ulcerative colitis (also known as *idiopathic proctocolitis*) and Crohn's disease (also known as *regional enteritis*). Both conditions are characterized by periods of acute exacerbations alternating with periods of remission.

The causes of IBD are not known, but infectious and autoimmune immunologic mechanisms are thought to play a part. Smoking is also associated with IBD.

Where It Occurs

- More common in whites than in blacks and Asians.
- Three to six times more common in people of Jewish heritage.
- Occurs slightly more often in women than in men.

Signal Symptoms

- Bloody stools, irregular bowel habits, passage of mucus.
- Tender colon, fever, sweats, malaise.
- Abdominal pain, cramping.

BE SAFE! Assess for signs of intestinal obstruction due to bowel inflammation and edema: cramping, bloating, pain, loud bowel sounds.

Diagnostic Tests

Test	What It Tells	Patient Problems/ Nursing Care
Colonoscopy	Visualizes bowel to allow for diagnosis	Knowledge deficit: explain procedures, including gastrointestinal prepping and NPO.

Treatment and Nursing Care

Potential Nursing Diagnoses*

Imbalanced nutrition, less than body requirements
Diarrhea
Disturbed body image
Anxiety

BE SMART! Provide a nutritional consultation to make sure the patient understands dietary modifications.

- Sulfasalazine is often prescribed in chronic cases with mild flare-ups. Mesalamine and other similar medications are used as anti-inflammatory agents. Antibiotics are used to treat infection.
- Patients are instructed to avoid foods that exacerbate symptoms.
- Surgical interventions, such as proctocolectomy with ileostomy, are also available. Surgery may be performed when patients fail to respond to conservative treatment.
- In acute situations, stop feedings, initiate nasogastric decompression, and begin IV fluid resuscitation along with electrolytes replacement and acid-base balance.
- Nursing care focuses on promoting physical and emotional comfort for the patient.

Intestinal Obstruction

Intestinal obstruction occurs when a blockage obstructs the normal flow of contents through the intestinal tract. Obstruction of the intestine causes the bowel to become vulnerable to ischemia. The intestinal mucosal barrier can be damaged, allowing intestinal bacteria to invade the intestinal wall and causing fluid exudation, which leads to hypovolemia and dehydration. About 7 L of fluid per day is secreted into the small intestine and stomach and usually reabsorbed. During obstruction, however, fluid accumulates, causing abdominal distention and pressure on the mucosal wall, which can lead to peritonitis and perforation. Obstructions can be partial or complete. The most common type of intestinal obstruction is one of the small intestine from fibrous adhesions.

The two major types of intestinal obstruction are mechanical and neurogenic (or nonmechanical). Neurogenic obstruction occurs primarily after manipulation of the bowel during surgery or with peritoneal irritation, pain of thoracolumbar origin, or intestinal ischemia. It is also caused by the effect of trauma or toxins on the nerves that regulate peristalsis, electrolyte imbalances, and neurogenic abnormalities such as spinal cord lesions. Mechanical obstruction of the bowel is caused by physical blockage of the intestine.

Where It Occurs

- Intestinal obstructions are more common in patients who have undergone major abdominal surgery or have congenital abnormalities of the bowel.
- When it occurs in a child, the obstruction is most likely to be an intussusception.
- Patients with irritable bowel syndrome, ulcerative colitis, Crohn's disease are at risk.

Signal Symptoms

- Cramping, bloating, pain, loud bowel sounds, abdominal distention.
- Signs of visible peristalsis or loops of large bowel may be observable.
- Dehydration: hypotension, tachycardia, dizziness, dry mouth, thirst.

BE SAFE! Infections should be treated promptly so that they do not progress to more serious conditions such as peritonitis and sepsis.

Diagnostic Tests

Test	What It Tells	Patient Problems/ Nursing Care
Chest and abdominal x-ray	Identifies free air under the diaphragm if perforation has occurred or blockage of lumen of bowel with distal passage of fluid and air (partial) or complete obstruction	Knowledge deficit: explain all procedures.
Water-soluble contrast enema	Identifies site and severity of colonic obstruction	Knowledge deficit: explain all procedures. Explain gastrointestinal prepping before test and NPO.

Treatment and Nursing Care

Potential Nursing Diagnoses*

Risk for infection

Fluid volume deficit

Imbalanced nutrition, less than body requirements

Pain (acute)

Diarrhea

Anxiety

BE SMART! Always auscultate the abdomen for up to 5 minutes for bowel sounds before palpation to make sure bowel sounds are present.

- Surgery is often indicated for a complete mechanical obstruction.
- Medical management with IV fluids, electrolytes, and administration of blood or plasma may be required for patients whose obstruction is caused by infection or inflammation or by a partial obstruction.
- Antibiotics may be prescribed when the obstruction is caused by an infectious process.
- Nursing care focuses on increasing the patient's comfort, postoperative management, and monitoring for complications.

Peptic Ulcer Disease

Peptic ulcer disease refers to ulcerative disorders in the lower esophagus, upper duodenum, and lower portion of the stomach. The types of peptic ulcers are gastric and duodenal, both of which are chronic diseases. The ulcer represents the development of a circumscribed defect in the gastric or duodenal mucosa that is exposed to acid and pepsin secretion. The ulcer may extend through the tissue layers of the muscle and serosa into the abdominal cavity. Stress ulcers, which are caused by a physiological response to major trauma, are clinically distinct from chronic peptic ulcers.

Gastric ulcers are less common than duodenal ulcers and usually occur in the lesser curvature of the stomach within 1 inch of the pylorus. The ulcer formation is caused by an inability of the mucosa to protect itself from damage by acid pepsin in the lumen (which is caused by a breakdown of the defensive factors). Duodenal ulcers occur in the proximal part of the duodenum (95%), are less than 1 cm in diameter, and are round or oval. A higher number of parietal cells in the stomach causes hypersecretion, or rapid emptying of the stomach; this may lead to a larger amount of acid being delivered to the first part of the duodenum and result in the formation of an ulcer.

Complications include obstruction, gastric cancer, fistula, and hemorrhage.

Where It Occurs

- The incidence of duodenal ulcers is highest in people 40 to 50 years old.
- Bleeding, anemia, early satiety, weight loss, dysphagia, nausea, vomiting.
- Family history of gastrointestinal cancer.

Signal Symptoms

- Nighttime pain, heartburn, chest discomfort, epigastric discomfort.
- Dyspepsia, including belching, bloating, and distention; fatty food intolerance.
- Pale mucous membranes and skin; anemia from acute or chronic blood loss.
- Some patients have black or tarry stools.

BE SAFE! Acute and chronic bleeding can lead to significant blood loss and hypovolemia.

Diagnostic Tests

Test	What It Tells	Patient Problems/ Nursing Care
Barium radiographic studies	Barium study highlights presence of ulcer in stomach or duodenum	Knowledge deficit: explain procedures, including gastrointestinal prepping and NPO.
Esophagogastroduodenoscopy	Flexible endoscopy to allow visualization of mucosa	Knowledge deficit: explain procedures, including gastrointestinal prepping and NPO.

Treatment and Nursing Care

Potential Nursing Diagnoses*

Pain (acute)
Fluid volume deficit
Fatigue
Diarrhea

BE SMART! Make sure patients understand their medications, the dose, route, and side effects.

- The treatment of choice for patients with peptic ulcers is generally pharmacologic.
- Proton pump inhibitors optimize ulcer healing by binding to the proton pump of parietal cells and inhibiting secretion of hydrogen ions into gastric lumen.
- Antibiotic therapy for *Helicobacter pylori* infection.
- H_2 antagonists reduce acid secretion to optimize ulcer healing.

- Diet restrictions are not necessary, but most specialists recommend only moderate alcohol use.
- Nurses should provide information about the cause and contributing factors as they pertain to the individual patient.

Peritonitis

Peritonitis is the inflammation of the serosal membrane of the peritoneal cavity and the organs within the cavity. The peritoneum is a double-layered, semipermeable, sterile sac that lines the abdominal cavity and covers all the organs in the abdominal cavity. Between its visceral and its parietal layers is the peritoneal cavity. Peritonitis can be sterile or infectious. Sterile peritonitis occurs when irritating substances such as bile, gastric acid, or foreign bodies are introduced into the cavity.

If a pathogen enters the peritoneum, an inflammatory response occurs. The most common cause is infection with *Escherichia coli*, but streptococci, staphylococci, and pneumococci may also cause the inflammation. Although the peritoneum walls off areas of contamination to prevent the spread of infection, if the contamination is massive or continuous, this defense mechanism may fail, resulting in peritonitis. If the infection continues, sepsis and septic shock can occur.

Where It Occurs

- Peritonitis can occur at any age and across both genders.
- The young adult male population is at risk because one of the primary causes of death in this gender and age group (multiple trauma) can lead to peritonitis.

Signal Symptoms

- Fever and chills, abdominal distention with rebound tenderness, guarding, and rigidity; pain increases with cough or movement.
- Diarrhea, nausea, paralytic ileus (abdominal distention, fullness, gas, cramping, constipation).
- Decreased bowel sounds, tachycardia, tachypnea.
- Late: Ascites, hypotension.

BE SAFE! Pain is severe. Discuss with health-care provider after the diagnosis is made which analgesics to use to manage pain.

Diagnostic Tests

Test	What It Tells	Patient Problems/ Nursing Care
White blood cell (WBC) count	Increased count indicates the presence of an infectious process	Knowledge deficit: explain procedures. Patient will need venipuncture.
Abdominal and chest x-rays	Inflammation leads to accumulation of fluid, perforation, or even rupture	Knowledge deficit: explain procedures.

Treatment and Nursing Care

Potential Nursing Diagnoses*

Pain (acute)
Risk for infection
Imbalanced nutrition, less than body requirements
Diarrhea
Knowledge deficit (medications, prevention, management)

BE SMART! Observe the patient for pallor, excessive sweating, or cold skin, which are signs of electrolyte and fluid loss. Respond quickly to peritonitis with antibiotic and fluid administration as prescribed.

- Interventions are supportive and include fluid and electrolyte replacement.
- If the peritonitis is caused by a perforation of the peritoneum, surgery is necessary as soon as the patient's condition is stabilized to eliminate the source of the infection by removing the foreign contents from the peritoneal cavity and inserting drains.
- Antibiotics halt the growth of bacteria and cause bacterial lysis.

- Analgesics relieve pain but can make diagnosis more difficult by masking changes in the patient's condition.
- Nursing care focuses on providing a stable, comfortable environment for the patient who is experiencing both physical and psychological stress.

Benign Prostatic Hypertrophy

Benign prostatic hyperplasia (BPH; excessive proliferation of normal cells in normal organs) or hypertrophy (an increase in size of an organ), one of the most common disorders of older men, is a nonmalignant enlargement of the prostate gland. It is the most common cause of obstruction of urine flow in men. The degree of enlargement determines whether or not bladder outflow obstruction occurs. As the urethra becomes obstructed, the muscle inside the bladder hypertrophies in an attempt to assist the bladder to force out the urine. BPH may also cause the formation of a bladder diverticulum that remains full of urine when the patient empties the bladder.

As the obstruction progresses, the bladder wall becomes thickened and irritable, and as it hypertrophies, it increases its own contractile force, leading to sensitivity even with small volumes of urine. Ultimately, the bladder gradually weakens and loses the ability to empty completely, leading to increased residual urine volume and urinary retention. With marked bladder distention, overflow incontinence may occur with any increase in intra-abdominal pressure such as that which occurs with coughing and sneezing. Because the condition occurs in older men, changes in hormone balances have been associated with the cause.

Where It Occurs

- By the age of 60, 50% of men have some degree of prostate enlargement, which is considered part of the normal aging process.
- As men become older, the incidence of symptoms increases to more than 75% for those over 80 years of age and 90% by 85 years of age.

Signal Symptoms

- Frequent urination, intermittent urination, nocturnal urination.
- Bladder distention may be present.
- Rubbery enlargement of the prostate found on digital exam indicates BPH; degree of enlargement does not consistently correlate with the degree of urinary obstruction.

BE SAFE! Urinary infections need to be treated promptly to avoid urosepsis.

Diagnostic Tests

Test	What It Tells	Patient Problems/ Nursing Care
Urinalysis, urine culture, blood culture	Urinary retention may lead to infection	Knowledge deficit: explain procedures. Patient may need venipuncture if blood infection is suspected. Do not contaminate specimens.
Uroflowmetry	Prostate inflammation leads to a narrowed urethral channel and obstruction of urine outflow	Knowledge deficit: explain procedures.

Treatment and Nursing Care

Potential Nursing Diagnoses*

Urinary retention
Risk for infection
Pain (acute)
Urinary elimination, impaired

BE SMART! Determine the amount of pain and discomfort associated with the digital exam.

- Those patients with the most severe cases, in which there is total urinary obstruction, chronic urinary retention, and recurrent urinary tract infection, usually require surgery, such as transurethral resection of the prostate (TURP).
- Phenoxybenzamine blocks effects of postganglionic synapses at the smooth muscle and exocrine glands.
- Finasteride shrinks prostate gland and improves urine flow.
- Antibiotics for positive urine or blood cultures.
- Nursing care may include assistance with catheter insertion and maintenance.

Cancer, Bladder

The majority of bladder tumors (>90%) are urothelial or transitional cell carcinomas arising in the epithelial layer of the bladder, although squamous cell (4%), adenocarcinoma (1% to 2%), and small cell (1%) may occur. Urothelial tumors are classified as invasive or noninvasive and, according to their shape, papillary or flat. Noninvasive urothelial cancer affects only the innermost layer of the bladder, whereas invasive urothelial cancer spreads from the urothelium to the deepest layers of the bladder. The deeper the invasion, the more serious the cancer. Papillary tumors have fingerlike projections that grow into the hollow of the bladder. Flat urothelial tumors involve the layer of cells closest to the inside of the bladder.

Most bladder tumors are multifocal, because the environment of the bladder allows for the continuous bathing of the mucosa with urine that contains tumor cells that can implant in several locations. The ureters, bladder neck, and prostate urethra may become obstructed. Direct extension can occur to the sigmoid colon, rectum, and depending on the sex of the patient, the prostate or uterus and vagina. Metastasis occasionally occurs to the bones, liver, and lungs. Bladder cancer is staged on the basis of the presence or absence of invasion and is graded (I to IV) on the basis of the degree of differentiation of the cell, with grade I being the best differentiated and slowest growing. The cause of bladder cancer is not well understood; however, cigarette smoking and occupational exposure to aromatic amines (textile dyes, rubber, hair dyes, paint pigment) are established risk factors.

Where It Occurs

- Bladder cancer occurs most frequently in persons over age 50, with more than half of the cases occurring in individuals over age 72.
- Bladder cancer is more common in men (1 in 30) than in women (1 in 90).
- Incidence is highest among European American men, with a rate twice that of African American men and four times that of European American women.
- Asians have the lowest incidence of bladder cancer.

Signal Symptoms

- Painless hematuria.
- Dysuria, urgency, or frequency of urination occur in 20% to 30% of patients with bladder cancer.
- The physical examination is usually normal.
- A bladder tumor becomes palpable only after extensive invasion into surrounding structures.

BE SAFE! Patients with bladder cancer need ongoing surveillance for reoccurrence for the first 3 years after treatment.

Diagnostic Tests

Test	What It Tells	Patient Problems/ Nursing Care
Cystoscopy/biopsy	Biopsy confirms the malignancy	Knowledge deficit: explain procedures.
Serum carcinoembryonic antigen (CEA) level	Approximately 50% of patients with late-stage bladder cancer have moderately elevated CEA levels	Knowledge deficit: explain procedures. Patient will need venipuncture.

Treatment and Nursing Care

Potential Nursing Diagnoses*

Impaired urinary elimination
Knowledge deficit (postoperative management, managing radiation therapy)
Pain (acute)
Ineffective coping
Risk for infection

BE SMART! Describe all drains, wounds, and drainage collection devices.

■ Patients with higher-stage invasive disease are usually treated with radical curative surgery, whereas patients with lower-stage noninvasive disease can be controlled with more conservative measures.

■ Intravesical chemotherapy reduces recurrence in those who had complete transurethral resection.

■ Stoma creation may be essential if radical cystectomy is done. Consultation with an enterostomal therapist will likely be needed.

■ Combination systemic chemotherapy may be effective in prolonging life but is rarely curative.

■ Postoperative patient education is essential.

Cancer, Prostate

Prostate cancer may begin with a condition called prostatic intraepithelial neoplasia (PIN), which can develop in men in their 20s. In this condition, there are microscopic changes in the size and shape of the prostate gland cells. The more abnormal the cells look, the more likely that cancer is present. It has been noted that 50% of men have PIN by the time they are 50 years old.

Adenocarcinomas compose 99% of the prostate cancers. They most frequently begin in the outer portion of the posterior lobe in the glandular cells of the prostate gland. Local spread occurs to the seminal vesicles, bladder, and peritoneum. Prostate cancer metastasizes to other sites via the hematologic and lymphatic systems, following a fairly predictable pattern. The pelvic and perivesicular lymph nodes and bones of the pelvis, sacrum, and lumbar spine are usually the first areas to be affected. Metastasis to other organs usually occurs late in the course of the disease, with the lungs, liver, and kidneys being most frequently involved. The cause of prostate cancer remains unclear, but age, viruses, family history, diet, and androgens are thought to have contributing roles.

Where It Occurs

- The peak incidence of prostate cancer is in men between ages 60 and 70; 85% of the cases are diagnosed in men over age 65.
- The highest incidence of prostate cancer occurs in African American men; Asians and Native Americans have the lowest rate.

Signal Symptoms

- Most men with early-stage prostate cancer are asymptomatic.
- Early-stage: nonraised, firm lesion of the prostate with a sharp edge; an advanced lesion is often hard and stonelike with irregular borders.

BE SAFE! Screening for prostate cancer is controversial; help male patients make informed decisions regarding screening.

Diagnostic Tests

Test	What It Tells	Patient Problems/ Nursing Care
Prostate-specific antigen (PSA)	The higher the level, the greater the tumor burden	Knowledge deficit: explain procedures. Patient will need venipuncture.
Transrectal ultrasound	Enlarged, solid prostate mass is noted	Knowledge deficit: explain procedures.

Treatment and Nursing Care

Potential Nursing Diagnoses*

Pain (chronic bone)
Ineffective sexuality pattern
Anxiety
Knowledge deficit (screening, sexual function, treatment options)

BE SMART! A suspicious prostatic mass is further evaluated by extending the examination to the groin to look for the presence of enlarged or tender lymph nodes.

■ Periodic observation, or "watchful waiting," may be proposed to a patient with early-stage, less-aggressive prostate cancer.
■ Radical prostatectomy has been the recommended treatment option for men with middle-stage disease because of high cure rates.
■ Both external beam radiotherapy and internal implant (brachytherapy) are used in the treatment of prostate cancer.
■ Analgesics are used to control pain.
■ Antineoplastics are used to treat or stabilize the disease.
■ Nursing care should include educating and explaining all procedures.

Chronic Renal Failure

Chronic renal failure (CRF) is irreversible renal dysfunction as manifested by the inability of the kidneys to excrete sufficient fluid and waste products from the body to maintain health. CRF is fatal if it is not treated. CRF is a progressive process; stages are defined by categorizing how much renal function remains. The first stage of renal deterioration is reduced renal reserve, which occurs when the patient has a glomerular filtration rate (GFR; the amount of filtrate formed by the kidneys each minute; normally 125 mL/min) of 35% to 50% of normal. The second stage, renal insufficiency, occurs when the patient has a GFR that is 25% to 35% of normal. The patient with renal failure has a GFR of 20% to 25% of normal. The patient with the final stage of renal dysfunction, end-stage renal disease (ESRD), has a GFR of 15% to 20% of normal or less.

All individuals with CRF experience similar physiological changes, regardless of the initial cause of the disease. The kidneys are unable to perform their normal functions of excretion of wastes, concentration of urine, regulation of blood pressure, regulation of acid-base balance, and production of erythropoietin (the hormone needed for red blood cell production and survival). CRF may be caused by either kidney disease or diseases of other systems.

Where It Occurs

■ Prevalence in various populations depends on predisposing conditions such as diabetes and hypertension; therefore, a significantly higher prevalence exists in the African American and Native American populations than in Asian Americans and whites.

■ CRF as a result of other diseases (diabetes mellitus or uncontrolled hypertension) is more common in the elderly simply because they have had the disease longer.

■ Medications such as aminoglycosides, sulfa, allopurinol can lead to CRF.

■ Vascular problems: renal artery stenosis, atheroemboli, hypertensive nephrosclerosis, renal vein thrombosis.

Signal Symptoms

■ Fatigue, nausea, vomiting, decreased libido, bleeding tendencies.

■ With potassium imbalance: rapid, irregular heart rates; distended jugular veins; and if pericarditis is present, a pericardial friction rub and distant heart sounds.

■ Respiratory symptoms: hyperventilation, Kussmaul breathing, dyspnea, orthopnea, and pulmonary congestion.

■ Late: urinelike odor on the breath and a yellow-gray cast to the skin.

BE SAFE! Observe for falls because patients may have difficulty with ambulation; they experience altered motor function and gait abnormalities, bone and joint pain, and peripheral neuropathy.

Diagnostic Tests

Test	What It Tells	Patient Problems/ Nursing Care
Blood urea nitrogen	Elevated levels indicate kidneys' inability to excrete waste	Knowledge deficit: explain procedures. Patient will need venipuncture.
Serum creatinine	Elevated levels indicate kidneys' inability to excrete waste	Knowledge deficit: explain procedures. Patient will need venipuncture.

Treatment and Nursing Care

Potential Nursing Diagnoses*

Fluid volume excess
Nausea
Activity intolerance
Impaired physical mobility
Knowledge deficit (medications, dialysis, nutrition)

> **BE SMART!** If patients are not candidates for renal transplantation, they must learn to live with renal failure their entire life. Patient education is critical.

- Patients who have progressed to ESRD require either dialysis or renal transplantation.
- Antihypertensives treat the underlying hypertension.
- Diuretics control fluid overload early in the disease if the patient is not anuric (total absence of urinary output).
- Patient education is critical. Patients must understand their medications, treatment options, nutritional needs, physical activity needs.

Glomerulonephritis

Acute glomerulonephritis (AGN) is an inflammatory disease of the specialized tuft of capillaries within the kidney called the *glomerulus*. The inflammatory changes occur because of deposits of antigen-antibody complexes lodged within the glomerular membrane. Antigen-antibody complexes are formed within the circulation in response to an antigen or foreign protein. The antigen may be of external origin, such as a portion of the streptococcus bacterial cell wall, or of internal origin, such as the changes that occur in systemic diseases like systemic lupus erythematosus (SLE).

If the source of the causative antigen is temporary, such as a transient infection, the inflammatory changes subside and renal function usually returns to normal; if the source of antigen is long term or permanent, the AGN may become chronic. During the acute phase of the disease process, major complications include hypertension, hypertensive encephalopathy, acute renal failure, cardiac failure, and seizures. Chronic glomerular nephritis leads to contracted, granular kidneys and end-stage renal disease. Rapidly progressive glomerulonephritis (RPGN; also known as *crescentic nephritis*), an acute and severe form of kidney inflammation, can cause loss of kidney function within days. Inflammation at the sites of renal filtration (the glomerular basement membrane) causes leakage of blood proteins into the urinary space. The condition is caused by inflammation of cells in the urinary space that form crescents, hence the name crescentic nephritis.

Where It Occurs

- AGN occurs primarily in the pediatric population, ages 5 to 15 years, after an infectious event
- RPGN primarily affects adults in their sixth and seventh decades of life.
- Twice as many males as females are affected with glomerulonephritis.

Signal Symptoms

- Decreased urine output; hematuria, dark, coffee-colored urine.
- Elevated blood pressure, fluid retention (edema in the face and hands), shortness of breath, azotemia (nausea, elevated blood urea nitrogen), headache, visual changes, seizures.

BE SAFE! During acute phases, control elevated blood pressure and fluid overload rapidly so that patient does not suffer ill effects.

Diagnostic Tests

Test	What It Tells	Patient Problems/ Nursing Care
Creatinine clearance	Damaged glomerulus no longer able to clear or filter normal amounts of creatinine from blood	Knowledge deficit: explain procedures. Patient will need venipuncture.
Serum creatinine	Decreased ability of glomerulus to filter creatinine leads to accumulation in the blood	Knowledge deficit: explain procedures. Patient will need venipuncture.

Treatment and Nursing Care

Potential Nursing Diagnoses*

Fluid volume excess
Nausea
Ineffective breathing pattern
Risk for infection
Nutrition imbalance, more than body requirements
Pain (acute)

BE SMART! Provide ongoing monitoring for visual changes, vomiting, adventitious breath sounds, abdominal distention, and seizure activity.

■ Most patients with AGN recover spontaneously.
■ Antihypertensive and diuretics manage hypertension and fluid overload. Angiotensin-converting enzyme (ACE) inhibitors may be given to patients with progressive disease.
■ Nurses focus on decreasing discomfort, reducing complications, and providing patient education with a focus on salt restriction, protein restriction, fluid volume control, and limiting infections.

Hemodialysis

Hemodialysis serves as an external kidney; blood flows through an external filter that removes extra fluid and wastes such as creatine and urea and is returned, cleansed, to the body. In patients with end-stage renal disease, hemodialysis occurs three times a week for 3 to 5 hours during each visit to a hemodialysis center, although nocturnal dialysis in the home is being studied. Three common ways are used to deliver hemodialysis: an intravenous catheter, an arteriovenous (AV) fistula, and a synthetic graft.

More than half a million patients with end-stage renal disease receive hemodialysis in the United States. Dialysis is associated with significant mortality, with approximately 30% of dialysis patients dying during the first year of treatment and an overall mortality rate of 20%. Complications from hemodialysis include anemia, sleep disorders, dialysis-related amyloidosis, itching, and renal osteodystrophy (bone disease of kidney failure).

Where It Occurs

- Older patients have the highest mortality rates when on dialysis.
- End-stage renal disease is more likely to occur in African Americans than in other races/ethnicities and is more common in men than in women.
- The highest prevalence in end-stage renal disease occurs in people over 65 years of age.

Signal Symptoms

- During the first months of dialysis: depression, fatigue; during dialysis, low blood pressure, headaches, and nausea.
- Serious, rare complications: bleeding, infection, sepsis, shock.

BE SAFE! Hyperkalemia (high potassium) is the most common cause of sudden death in dialysis patients and usually occurs when patients miss their treatments.

Diagnostic Tests

No specific tests are appropriate for hemodialysis. Because bleeding and infection are both possible complications, generally patients have blood chemistries and complete blood count obtained periodically after dialysis.

Treatment and Nursing Care

Potential Nursing Diagnoses*

Risk for infection
Fluid volume deficit
Nutrition, imbalanced, less than body requirements
Nausea
Anxiety

BE SMART! Assess the dialysis access port (an IV catheter, an AV fistula, and a synthetic graft) for signs of bleeding, irritation, or infection.

■ Assess the vascular access before and after each dialysis session. Teach the patient how to clean the site and to observe for signs of infection.
■ Provide patient education on the importance of attending the dialysis sessions and on the type, dose, and side effects of all medications.
■ Monitor vital signs carefully for signs of excessive bleeding or shock.
■ Assess the patient for signs of complications.

Hydronephrosis

Hydronephrosis is the distention of the pelvis and calyces of one or both kidneys, resulting in thinning of the renal tubules because of obstructed urinary flow. When the obstruction is a stone or kink in one of the ureters, only one kidney is damaged. The obstruction causes backup, resulting in increased pressure in the kidneys. If the pressure is low to moderate, the kidney may dilate with no obvious loss of function.

Over time, intermittent or continuous high pressure causes irreversible nephron destruction. If the patient has a chronic partial obstruction, the kidneys lose their ability to concentrate urine. The kidneys may lose renal mass and atrophy and have a lowered resistance to infection and pyelonephritis because of urinary stasis. If hydronephrosis is caused by an acute obstructive uropathy (any disease of the urinary tract), the patient may develop a paralytic ileus. If bilateral hydronephrosis is left untreated, renal failure can result.

Where It Occurs

■ Men 60 years of age and older with prostate difficulties have a higher risk of hydronephrosis than women of the same age.
■ Urinary tract obstruction is rare in children.

Signal Symptoms

■ Asymmetry in the flank area indicates the presence of a renal mass.
■ Urinary retention, fever, pain, hematuria.
■ Inspection of the male urethra may reveal stenosis, injury, or phimosis.

BE SAFE! A genitourinary (GU) examination is performed in the female patient to inspect and palpate for vaginal, uterine, and rectal lesions.

Diagnostic Tests

Test	What It Tells	Patient Problems/ Nursing Care
Ultrasonography	Distention of the renal pelvis and calyces results from obstruction of urine outflow	Knowledge deficit: explain procedures.
Serum creatinine	Decreased ability of glomerulus to filter creatinine leads to accumulation in the blood	Knowledge deficit: explain procedures. Patient will need venipuncture.

Treatment and Nursing Care

Potential Nursing Diagnoses*

Impaired urinary elimination
Risk for infection
Fluid volume excess
Pain (acute)

BE SMART! A distended bladder may indicate urinary retention and obstruction.

- Temporary urinary drainage may be achieved by a nephrostomy or ureterostomy.
- Antibiotics are prescribed to manage bacterial infections.
- Analgesics relieve pain.
- Nursing care should focus on maintaining drainage of urinary system and monitoring fluid balance.

Nephrolithiasis

Nephrolithiasis, or renal calculi, is the formation of stones in the kidneys from the crystallization of minerals and other substances that normally dissolve in the urine. Renal calculi vary in size, with 90% of them smaller than 5 mm in diameter; some, however, grow large enough to prevent the natural passage of urine through the ureter. Calculi may be solitary or multiple. Approximately 80% of these stones are composed of calcium salts. Other types are the struvite stones (which contain magnesium, ammonium, and phosphate), uric acid stones, and cystine stones. If the calculi remain in the renal pelvis or enter the ureter, they can damage renal parenchyma (functional tissue). Larger calculi can cause pressure necrosis. In certain locations, calculi cause obstruction, lead to hydronephrosis, and tend to recur.

The precise cause of nephrolithiasis is unknown, although they are associated with dehydration, urinary obstruction, calcium levels, and other factors.

Where It Occurs

- Nephrolithiasis occurs more often in men than in women, unless heredity is a factor, and occurs most often between ages 30 and 50 years.
- The prevalence is higher in whites and people of Asian ancestry than in other populations.
- Associated conditions: low fluid intake, excess dietary calcium intake, overactive calcium absorption mechanisms.

Signal Symptoms

- Severe and excruciating, intense pain; often flank pain radiating to the groin; inability to find a comfortable position.
- Percussion of the costovertebral angle elicits severe pain.
- Hematuria, fever, malaise, fatigue, nausea, vomiting.

BE SAFE! Monitor the patient for signs of an infection such as fever, chills, and increased white blood cell counts.

Diagnostic Tests

Test	What It Tells	Patient Problems/ Nursing Care
Helical computed tomography scan without contrast	Visualizes size, shape, relative position of stone	Knowledge deficit: explain procedures.
Kidney-ureter-bladder and abdominal x-rays	Reveals most renal calculi except cystine and uric acid stones	Knowledge deficit: explain procedures.

Treatment and Nursing Care

Potential Nursing Diagnoses*

Pain (acute)
Impaired urinary elimination
Risk for infection
Fluid volume deficit
Nausea

BE SMART! Correct fluid volume deficit and infection.

- Nephrolithiasis can be treated with surgical removal or vigorous hydration that can be supplemented with active medical expulsive therapy.
- Analgesia relaxes the ureter and facilitates the passage of a stone. The pain is severe and needs to be treated with IV opioids.
- Some physicians will request that all urine be strained to locate any stones that are expelled.
- Observe for urinary obstruction: abdominal distention, pain, anuria, nausea, and vomiting progressing to renal failure.
- Nursing care focuses on fluid replacement, managing infection and hematuria, and educating the patient on medications and prevention.

Neurogenic Bladder

Neurogenic bladder is an interruption of normal bladder innervation because of lesions on or insults to the nervous system. Neurogenic bladder dysfunctions are categorized in two ways: according to the response of the bladder to the insult (classification I) or according to the lesion's level (classification II). Insult classifications include uninhibited, sensory paralytic, motor paralytic, autonomous, and reflex. Lesion-level classifications include upper motor neuron damage and lower motor neuron damage.

Causes include brain lesion (stroke, brain tumor, Parkinson's disease) spinal cord lesion (multiple sclerosis, spinal cord injury), and peripheral nerve injury (polio, Guillain-Barré syndrome). Complications include urinary retention, urinary urgency, infection, incontinence.

Where It Occurs

■ The incidence and manifestations of neurogenic bladder dysfunction do not change with age, and there are no known specific racial or ethnic considerations.

Signal Symptoms

■ With spastic neurogenic bladder, the patient may have increased anal sphincter tone so that when you touch the abdomen, thigh, or genitalia, the patient may void spontaneously.
■ Pain, urinary urgency, bladder distention, urinary incontinence, residual urine in the bladder even after voiding.
■ Fever, malaise, weakness, fatigue, cloudy or foul-smelling urine.
■ For flaccid neurogenic bladder, palpate and percuss the bladder to evaluate for a distended bladder; usually, the patient will not sense bladder fullness despite large bladder distention because of sensory deficits.

BE SAFE! In patients with urinary incontinence, evaluate the groin and perineal area for skin irritation and breakdown.

Diagnostic Tests

Test	What It Tells	Patient Problems/ Nursing Care
Uroflowmetry	Completeness and speed of bladder emptying are both reduced	Knowledge deficit: explain procedures. Use sterile technique to prevent infection.
Cystometry	Evaluates detrusor muscle function and tonicity, determines etiology of bladder dysfunction, and differentiates among classifications of bladder dysfunction	Knowledge deficit: explain procedures. Use sterile technique to prevent infection.

Treatment and Nursing Care

Potential Nursing Diagnoses*

Impaired urinary elimination
Pain (acute)
Risk for infection
Urinary incontinence, overflow
Urinary retention

BE SMART! If urinary drainage is initiated, protect the patient from infection. Generally 500 to 750 cc are drained at one time from the bladder, the catheter is clamped for a set period of time (sometimes 2 hours), and then another 500 to 750 is drained.

■ If all attempts at bladder retraining or catheterization have failed, a surgeon may perform a reconstructive procedure.
■ Alpha-adrenergic drugs contract the bladder neck and thereby increase bladder outlet resistance.

- Antimuscarinic (anticholinergic) drugs decrease spasticity and incontinence in spastic neurogenic bladder disorders. Patients may be placed on antibiotics to treat or prevent infection.
- Nurses should focus on bladder training or catheter care. Teach the patient how to prevent infection and to maintain adequate drainage.

Pheochromocytoma

Pheochromocytoma is a rare tumor, most often located in the adrenal gland, that arises from catecholamine-producing chromaffin cells. These tumors secrete large quantities of epinephrine and norepinephrine, resulting in persistent or paroxysmal hypertension. Pheochromocytomas are vascular tumors that contain hemorrhagic or cystic areas and are most often well encapsulated, with 90% of the tumors being benign. The tumors are generally less than 6 cm in diameter and usually weigh less than 100 g.

Some 80% of these tumors arise from the adrenal medulla and are unilateral. These tumors follow the rule of 10s: 10% occur in children, 10% are bilateral or multiple, 10% are familial, 10% are malignant, 10% recur after surgical removal, and 10% are extra-adrenal. The 10% located in extra-adrenal sites are known as *paragangliomas*. Complications include cerebrovascular accident, retinopathy, heart disease, metastatic cancer, and renal failure. Patients with pheochromocytoma are also at higher risk for complications during operative procedures, pregnancy, and diagnostic testing. Most patients develop a pheochromocytoma from unknown causes.

Where It Occurs

- Pheochromocytoma occurs equally in men and women, has no racial or ethnic predominance, and most commonly occurs between the ages of the early 20s and the late 50s.
- There are links to family ancestry in pheochromocytoma predisposition.

Signal Symptoms

- Headache, diaphoresis, weakness, fatigue, tremor, flushing.
- Persistent blood elevation pressure with orthostatic hypotension.

- Nausea, impending sense of doom, anxiety, palpitation.
- Epigastric pain, flank pain, constipation.

BE SAFE! Although pheochromocytoma occurs in only 0.1% to 0.3% of all hypertensive patients, hypertension may be fatal if the pheochromocytoma goes unrecognized.

Diagnostic Tests

Test	What It Tells	Patient Problems/ Nursing Care
Computed tomography scan or magnetic resonance imaging	Identifies location and size of tumor	Knowledge deficit: explain procedures.
Free urine catecholamines, vanillylmandelic acid (VMA) and metanephrines (24 hr)	Elevated amount of catecholamines are excreted in the urine	Knowledge deficit: explain procedures.

Treatment and Nursing Care

Potential Nursing Diagnoses*

Risk for injury
Pain (acute)
Anxiety
Fear
Knowledge deficit (treatment options, medications, pathophysiology)

BE SMART! Postoperatively, hypovolemic shock and hypotension are critical concerns because of the rapid decrease in circulating catecholamines.

- More than 90% of pheochromocytomas can be cured by surgical removal, and patients who do not have operative tumors are treated pharmacologically.
- Alpha-adrenergic blocking agents are used preoperatively to control blood pressure and prevent intraoperative hypertensive crisis.

- Beta-adrenergic blockers manage hypertension for patients with a heart rate greater than 110, history of dysrhythmias, or epinephrine-secreting tumor.
- Nursing care should focus on monitoring blood pressure and discussing treatment options.

Polycystic Kidney Disease

Although inherited polycystic diseases are not the only types of cystic diseases of the kidney, all types are a major contributor to chronic renal failure. Infantile autosomal recessive polycystic kidney disease (RPKD) and autosomal dominant polycystic kidney disease (ADPKD) are two types of inherited polycystic kidney disease. Infantile (RPKD) disease affects both kidneys, leads to renal failure, and causes biliary dilation and fibrosis in the liver. The basic pathology of cyst development is a weakening of the basement membrane, which possibly is caused by an abnormality of the extracellular connective tissue cells. Adult-onset disease (ADPKD) is a bilateral disorder, although it may have asymmetrical progression with multiple expanding cysts that destroy renal function. Renal deterioration eventually leads to uremia, chronic renal failure, and the need for chronic renal dialysis. ADPKD has a genetic origin.

Where It Occurs

- RPKD always becomes apparent during childhood in boys and girls, usually before age 13.
- Most adult patients with ADPKD are identified between ages 30 and 50 years.

Signal Symptoms

- Dilute urine due to decreased concentrating ability, albuminuria, hypertension, flank pain, hematuria.
- Cloudy, foul-smelling urine.
- Infants with RPKD: pronounced epicanthal folds, a pointed nose and small chin, and low-set ears.

BE SAFE! Treat all urinary infections promptly to conserve renal function.

Diagnostic Tests

Test	What It Tells	Patient Problems/ Nursing Care
Genetic testing	Genetic alterations lead to ADPKD	Knowledge deficit: explain procedures. Patient will need venipuncture.
Renal ultrasound	Cyst development leads to altered tubular epithelium, cell proliferation, and fluid secretion	Knowledge deficit: explain procedures.

Treatment and Nursing Care

Potential Nursing Diagnoses*

Pain (acute)
Risk for infection
Impaired urinary elimination
Risk for fluid balance imbalance

BE SMART! Talk with parents about the potential results of genetic testing and refer them to a genetics counselor.

- Because there is no cure for polycystic kidney disease, care centers around alleviating symptoms and slowing the onset of renal impairment.
- Medications are administered to manage hypertension, infection, renal insufficiency, and end-stage renal disease.
- Analgesic drugs may be needed for control of the flank pain associated with enlarged kidneys.
- One of the most important nursing roles is to promote the patient's comfort, along with managing treatment decisions and monitoring dialysis or transplant.

Pyelonephritis

Pyelonephritis is an infection of the renal pelvis and renal tissue by invasion of microorganisms. It can be either acute (also known as *acute infective tubulointerstitial nephritis*) or chronic in nature, as differentiated by the clinical picture and long-term effects. The infection, which primarily affects the renal pelvis, calyces, and medulla, progresses through the urinary tract as organisms ascend the ureters from the bladder because of vesicoureteral reflux (reflux of urine up the ureter during micturition) or contamination.

Acute pyelonephritis occurs 24 to 48 hours after contamination of the urethra or after instrumentation such as a catheterization. Acute pyelonephritis is potentially life threatening and often causes scarring of the kidney with each infection. Complications include calculus formation, renal abscesses, renal failure, septic shock, and chronic pyelonephritis. Chronic pyelonephritis is a persistent infection that causes progressive inflammation and scarring. It usually occurs after chronic obstruction or because of vesicoureteral reflux. This destruction of renal cells may alter the urine-concentrating capability of the kidney and can lead to chronic renal failure.

Where It Occurs

- Pyelonephritis occurs more often in women than in men because the female urethra is much shorter than the male urethra.
- The incidence of pyelonephritis is highest in white females, and in particular adolescent and young adult females who are sexually active.

Signal Symptoms

- Urinary frequency, hesitancy, and urgency; lower abdominal pain.
- Percussion or deep palpation over the costovertebral angle elicits marked tenderness.
- Urine with abnormal color, cloudiness, blood, or presence of a foul odor.
- Low-grade temperature, fatigue, weakness.

BE SAFE! If infection is not treated promptly, sepsis and septic shock may follow.

Diagnostic Tests

Test	What It Tells	Patient Problems/ Nursing Care
Urine culture and sensitivity	Identifies bacterial contaminants	Knowledge deficit: explain all procedures.
Urinalysis	Shows the presence of white blood cells and pus	Knowledge deficit: explain all procedures.

Treatment and Nursing Care

Potential Nursing Diagnoses*

Risk for infection
Pain (acute)
Impaired urinary elimination
Urinary retention

BE SMART! Hypertension is common in patients with chronic pyelonephritis and needs to be controlled with medication.

- The goal of therapy is to rid the urinary tract of the pathogenic organisms and to relieve an obstruction if present.
- Surgery is performed only if an underlying defect is causing obstruction, reflux, or calculi.
- Antibiotics eradicate bacteria and maintain adequate blood levels.
- Nurses should provide comfort for patient with flank pain, headache, and irritating urinary tract symptoms.

Renal Calculi

Nephrolithiasis is the formation of renal calculi (kidney stones) from the crystallization of minerals and other substances that normally dissolve in the urine. Renal calculi vary in size, with 90% of them smaller than 5 mm in diameter; some, however, grow large enough to prevent the natural passage of urine through the ureter. Calculi may be solitary or multiple. Approximately 80% of these stones are composed of calcium salts. Other types are the struvite stones (which contain magnesium, ammonium, and phosphate), uric acid stones, and cystine stones. If the calculi remain in the renal pelvis or enter the ureter, they can damage renal parenchyma (functional tissue). Larger calculi can cause pressure necrosis. In certain locations, calculi cause obstruction, lead to hydronephrosis, and tend to recur.

The precise cause of nephrolithiasis is unknown, although they are associated with dehydration, urinary obstruction, calcium levels, and other factors.

Where It Occurs

- Nephrolithiasis occurs more often in men than in women, unless heredity is a factor, and occurs most often between ages 30 and 50 years.
- The prevalence is higher in whites and people of Asian ancestry than in other populations.
- Associated conditions: low fluid intake, excess dietary calcium intake, overactive calcium absorption mechanisms.

Signal Symptoms

- Severe and excruciating, intense pain; often flank pain radiating to the groin; inability to find a comfortable position.
- Percussion of the costovertebral angle elicits severe pain.
- Hematuria, fever, malaise, fatigue, nausea, vomiting.

BE SAFE! Monitor the patient for signs of an infection such as fever, chills, and increased white blood cell counts.

Diagnostic Tests

Test	What It Tells	Patient Problems/ Nursing Care
Helical computed tomography scan without contrast	Visualizes size, shape, relative position of stone	Knowledge deficit: explain procedures.
Kidney-ureter-bladder and abdominal x-rays; renal sonogram	Reveals most renal calculi except cystine and uric acid stones	Knowledge deficit: explain procedures.

Treatment and Nursing Care

Potential Nursing Diagnoses*

Pain (acute)
Impaired urinary elimination
Risk for infection
Fluid volume deficit
Nausea

BE SMART! Correct fluid volume deficit and infection.

- Nephrolithiasis can be treated with surgical removal or vigorous hydration that can be supplemented with active medical expulsive therapy.
- Analgesia relaxes the ureter and facilitates the passage of a stone. The pain is severe and needs to be treated with IV opioids.
- Some physicians will request that all urine be strained to locate any stones that are expelled.
- Observe for urinary obstruction: abdominal distention, pain, anuria, nausea, and vomiting progressing to renal failure.
- Nursing care focuses on fluid replacement, managing infection and hematuria, and educating the patient on medications and prevention.

Renal Failure

Acute renal failure (ARF) is the abrupt deterioration of renal function that results in the accumulation of fluids, electrolytes, and metabolic waste products. It is usually accompanied by a marked decrease in urinary output. Although ARF is often reversible, if it is ignored or inappropriately treated, it can lead to irreversible kidney damage and chronic renal failure. Two types of ARF occur: community- and hospital-acquired. Community-acquired ARF is diagnosed in about 1% of hospital admissions at the time of initial assessment. In comparison, hospital-acquired ARF occurs in up to 4% of hospital admissions and 20% of critical care admissions. ARF can be classified as prerenal (due to poor circulation or hypovolemia), intra-renal (due to toxic chemicals, glomerular damage, or renal ischemia), and postrenal (due to obstruction in the bladder or urethra).

Approximately 70% of patients develop oliguric ARF with a urine output of less than 500 mL/day. The other 30% of patients never develop oliguria and have what is considered nonoliguric renal failure. Oliguric ARF generally has three stages. During the initial phase (often called the oliguric phase), when trauma or insult affects the kidney tissue, the patient becomes oliguric. This stage may last a week or more. The second stage of ARF is the diuretic phase, which is heralded by a doubling of the urinary output from the previous 24 hours. During the diuretic phase, patients may produce as much as 5 L of urine in 24 hours but lack the ability for urinary concentration and regulation of waste products. This phase can last from 1 to several weeks. The final stage, the recovery phase, is characterized by a return to a normal urinary output (about 1,500 to 1,800 mL/24 hr), with a gradual improvement in metabolic waste removal. Some patients take up to a year to recover full renal function after the initial insult. The following conditions are associated with acute renal failure: hypertension, heart failure, multiple myeloma, chronic infection, exposure to chemicals such as ethyl alcohol or ethylene glycol, mercury, lead, cadmium, and certain antibiotics and chemotherapeutic agents.

Where It Occurs

- The elderly are more susceptible to insults that result in ARF.
- There are no known racial or ethnic considerations.

Signal Symptoms

- General: drowsiness, irritability, confusion due to the accumulation of metabolic wastes.
- Oliguric phase: fluid overload, hypertension, rapid heart rate, peripheral edema, and crackles.
- Diuretic phase: dehydration, with dry mucous membranes, poor skin turgor, flat neck veins, and orthostatic hypotension.
- Prerenal: thirst, dehydration, low urine output, dizziness, orthostatic hypotension.
- Intrarenal: hematuria, edema, hypertension.
- Postrenal: urgency, frequency, hesitancy.

BE SAFE! When the kidneys cannot clear body wastes, all organ systems are involved, including respiratory (generally rapid respiratory rate to manage metabolic acidosis), cardiac (tachycardia), gastrointestinal (nausea, vomiting), and central nervous system (irritability).

Diagnostic Tests

Test	What It Tells	Patient Problems/ Nursing Care
Urinalysis	Acute damage to kidneys causes loss of red and white blood cells, casts (fibrous material or coagulated protein), or protein in the urine	Knowledge deficit: explain all procedures.
Blood urea nitrogen and serum creatinine	Kidneys cannot excrete wastes, so levels are elevated	Knowledge deficit: explain all procedures. Patient will need venipuncture.

Treatment and Nursing Care

Potential Nursing Diagnoses*

Fluid volume imbalance
Impaired urinary elimination
Nausea
Fatigue
Imbalanced nutrition

BE SMART! Patients need teaching about fluid balance, activity, and nutrition until the kidneys regain their function.

■ Electrolyte replacement is based on the patient's serum electrolyte values.
■ Renal replacement therapy includes intermittent hemodialysis (IHD), continuous venovenous hemodiafiltration (CVVHD), and peritoneal dialysis (PD).

- Diuretics convert oliguric ARF to nonoliguric.
- Low-dose dopamine is a potent vasodilator, increasing renal blood flow and urine output.
- Rest and recovery are important nursing goals.

TURP

Transurethral resection of the prostate (TURP) is the primary surgical treatment for obstructive prostatic hypertrophy. Benign prostatic hyperplasia (BPH), or benign prostatic hypertrophy, occurs with proliferation of the cellular elements of the prostate. It is one of the most common disorders of older men, a nonmalignant enlargement of the prostate gland, and the most common cause of obstruction of urine flow in men. The degree of enlargement determines whether or not bladder outflow obstruction occurs. As the urethra becomes obstructed, the muscle inside the bladder hypertrophies in an attempt to assist the bladder to force out the urine. BPH may also cause the formation of a bladder diverticulum that remains full of urine when the patient empties the bladder.

TURP allows the surgeon to remove prostate tissue using minimally invasive surgical techniques. The surgeon inserts a resectoscope through the penis. The surgeon controls irrigating fluid and an electrical loop that cuts tissue one slice at a time and then seals blood vessels. The irrigation fluid carries the slices into the bladder, and then they are flushed out of the bladder through a catheter at the end of the operation. Complications include infection, urinary obstruction, and hemorrhage.

Where It Occurs

- TURP is used to manage obstructive prostatic hypertrophy when medical therapy with 5-alpha reductase inhibitors, alpha-adrenergic blockers, and prostatic growth inhibitors do not reduce or moderate prostate growth and symptoms of obstruction (urinary retention).
- Generally performed in males, 60 to 80 years of age (average age about 69 years).
- African American men generally have more complicating medical conditions than other populations.

Signal Symptoms

- Urinary retention.
- Urinary tract infections: foul-smelling or cloudy urine, hematuria, dysuria; fever, suprapubic or flank tenderness, malaise, fatigue; urinary retention, urgency, frequency due to prostatic hypertrophy.

BE SAFE! Check the drainage system and keep it free flowing and unobstructed by blood clots and kinks.

Diagnostic Tests

Test	What It Tells	Patient Problems/ Nursing Care
Complete blood count	Presence of bleeding or infection	Knowledge deficit: explain procedures. Patient will need venipuncture.
Filling cystometry and bladder pressure-flow studies	Identifies presence or absence of urinary retention	Knowledge deficit: explain procedures.

Treatment and Nursing Care

Potential Nursing Diagnoses*

Pain (acute)
Risk for infection
Risk for fluid volume deficit
Ineffective sexuality pattern

BE SMART! Monitor fluid and electrolyte balance, especially hyponatremia, because of irrigation solution; signs and symptoms include disorientation, nausea, vomiting, fatigue, and even brain edema and seizures.

- Generally spinal anesthesia is performed for the TURP.
- The surgeon removes the obstructing tissue while minimizing damage to surrounding structures using luminal prostate resection with cystoscopic procedures (electrosurgical TURP).
- Teach patient to (1) avoid straining, especially during bowel movements; (2) avoid lifting heavy objects; (3) drink fluids.
- Explain when follow-up appointments are scheduled. Teach signs of urinary obstruction, infection, hemorrhage. Teach about all antibiotics.

Urinary Tract Infection

Urinary tract infections (UTIs) are common and usually occur because of the entry of bacteria into the urinary tract at the urethra. Urinary reflux is one reason that bacteria spread in the urinary tract. Vesicourethral reflux occurs when pressure increases in the bladder from coughing or sneezing and pushes urine into the urethra. When pressure returns to normal, the urine moves back into the bladder, taking with it bacteria from the urethra.

In vesicoureteral reflux, urine flows backward from the bladder into one or both of the ureters, carrying bacteria from the bladder to the ureters and widening the infection. If they are left untreated, UTIs can lead to chronic infections, pyelonephritis, and even systemic sepsis and septic shock. If infection reaches the kidneys, permanent renal damage can occur, which leads to acute and chronic renal failure. The pathogen that accounts for about 90% of UTIs is *Escherichia coli*.

Where It Occurs

- Women are more prone than men to UTIs because of natural anatomic variations.
- Incidence increases with age, especially once sexual activity begins.

Signal Symptoms

- Urinary frequency, hesitancy, and urgency; lower abdominal pain.
- Percussion or deep palpation over the costovertebral angle elicits marked tenderness.

- Urine with abnormal color, cloudiness, blood, or presence of a foul odor.
- Low-grade temperature, fatigue, weakness.

BE SAFE! Surveillance for sexually transmitted infections is recommended as part of the examination.

Diagnostic Tests

Test	What It Tells	Patient Problems/ Nursing Care
Leukocyte esterase dip test	Presence of leukocyte esterase indicates UTI	Knowledge deficit: explain all procedures.
Urine culture and sensitivity	Identifies causative organism	Knowledge deficit: explain all procedures.

Treatment and Nursing Care

Potential Nursing Diagnoses*

Impaired urinary elimination
Risk for infection
Pain (acute)
Knowledge deficit (medications, prevention, pain management)

BE SMART! Encourage patient to take entire course of antibiotics.

- An acid-ash diet may be encouraged.
- Cephalosporins and ciprofloxacin (Cipro) are two bacteriocidals prescribed, depending on the invading organism.
- Nurses should encourage patients with infections to increase fluid intake to promote frequent urination.

Cancer, Bone

Bone cancers are sarcomas—that is, cancers of connective tissue. Primary bone cancers are relatively uncommon. Most (60%–65%) tumors of the bone are secondary, or metastatic, ones from other primary tumors. Cancers originating in the osseous, cartilaginous (chondrogenic), or membrane tissue are classified as bone cancer. Cancers originating from the bone marrow are usually classified as hematologic cancers.

The most common type of primary bone cancer is osteosarcoma. Osteosarcoma and chondrosarcoma are the most common sarcomas of the bone and comprise 70% of all bone cancers. The remainder of bone cancers are Ewing's sarcoma, chordomas, and malignant histiocytoma and fibrosarcomas. Evidence links the development of bone cancer with exposure to therapeutic radiation.

Where It Occurs

- Primary cancers of the bone are more common in males and tend to occur in the late teen years or after age 60.
- Incidence of osteosarcoma is slightly higher in African Americans than in whites.

Signal Symptoms

- Dull aching pain.
- Inability to move a joint or weakness of the affected limb.
- If the tumor has progressed, weight loss or cachexia, fever, and decreased mobility may be noted.

BE SAFE! Protect the patient from falls by surveying the environment and providing mobility assistance when needed.

Diagnostic Tests

Test	What It Tells	Patient Problems/ Nursing Care
Serum alkaline phosphatase	Elevations occur with formation of new bone by increasing osteoblastic activity	Knowledge deficit: explain procedures. Patient will need venipuncture.
X-rays and computed tomography (CT)	CT shows extent of soft tissue damage and provides a visualization of the lesions	Knowledge deficit: explain procedures.

Treatment and Nursing Care

Potential Nursing Diagnoses*

Impaired physical mobility
Pain (acute, chronic)
Risk for infection
Risk for falls
Knowledge deficit (postoperative care)

BE SMART! Begin physical rehabilitation as soon after surgery as indicated to maintain muscle tone and prevent edema.

- Radiation has variable effectiveness in bone cancer.
- Surgery may range from simple curettage, when primary bone cancer is confined, to amputation or extensive resection such as a leg amputation with hemipelvectomy.
- Chemotherapy is often used preoperatively to reduce the size of the tumor or postoperatively to help eliminate the risk of micrometastasis.
- Nursing care should focus on postoperative care or management of other treatment methods.

Compartment Syndrome

Compartment syndrome (CS) generally occurs with injury to the extremities. After injury, tissue pressure within a closed muscle compartment increases above the pressure needed to allow for the circulation of blood. With no blood supply to the muscles and nerves, tissue ischemia occurs and, if now rapidly reversed, tissue death follows. Causes include trauma, bone fractures, exercise, limb compression, bleeding, thrombosis, and (rarely) intramuscular injection.

Where It Occurs

■ Chronic exertional CS occurs in athletes when they have repetitive loading or exertional exercise that traumatize the extremities, and it occurs particularly in the legs.
■ CS is found in up to 10% of leg fractures.

Signal Symptoms

■ Pain out of proportion to the injury; feelings of tightness.
■ Decreased blood flow and accumulation of wastes leads to pain, decreased sensation, swelling, pallor, and decreased capillary blanching.
■ Late signs: faint or absent peripheral pulses, hypoesthesia (partial loss of sensation), paresis (slight or partial paralysis), extremities necrosis.

BE SAFE! CS needs rapid action so that tissue ischemia and death does not occur.

Diagnostic Tests

Test	What It Tells	Patient Problems/ Nursing Care
Measurement of compartment pressure	Determines compartment pressure; generally 30–45 mm Hg at rest is considered diagnostic for CS	Knowledge deficit: explain procedures.

Treatment and Nursing Care

Potential Nursing Diagnoses*

Ineffective tissue perfusion (peripheral)
Pain (acute)
Risk for infection
Risk for injury

BE SMART! If the patient receives a fasciotomy, observe the surgical site for bleeding and infection.

- Conservative management: rest, water exercises, massage, stretching.
- Fasciotomy (surgical procedure in which surgeon cuts fascia, or fibrous tissue, to relieve tension or pressure) followed by physical therapy program to regain function, limited weight bearing, crutches.
- Patient teaching: medications, prevention of infection, activity levels.

Hip Fracture

Hip fractures most commonly occur in the elderly population as a result of a fall from a standing height. In younger patients, such fractures are most commonly the result of motor vehicle crashes or injuries related to athletic activities. Hip fractures are classified according to their relation to the hip capsule, location, and extent of displacement. Risk factors include cigarette smoking, physical inactivity, alcohol misuse, institutional living, maternal history of hip fracture, general cardiovascular disease, and poor vision. In addition, hip fractures are associated with antipsychotic medications and protease inhibitor therapy for HIV infection.

Where It Occurs

- Incidence increases with age.
- Whites are two to three times more likely than non-whites to suffer a hip fracture.
- Females are more likely than males to suffer a hip fracture.
- Approximately 20% of patients die in the year after a hip fracture, likely because of complications from immobility.

Signal Symptoms

- Pain, inability to move the hip, misalignment of legs.
- In young patients with athletic injuries, pain may be in the hip or knee.
- Patients may have other injuries, such as extremity injuries, intra-abdominal or intrapelvic injuries, neck injuries, and head injuries.

BE SAFE! Watch for signs of shock; hip fractures are associated with as much as 1,500 cc of blood loss.

Diagnostic Tests

Test	What It Tells	Patient Problems/ Nursing Care
Hip x-rays	Demonstrates radiographic evidence of injury	Knowledge deficit: explain all procedures.

Treatment and Nursing Care

Potential Nursing Diagnoses*

Fluid volume deficit
Pain (acute)
Risk for injury
Mobility, bed, impaired
Knowledge deficit (medications, pain relief, mobility)

BE SMART! Prevention is important. Assess older patients' gait and home environment to reduce the risk of falls and hip fractures.

- Surgical intervention for femoral neck fractures, intertrochanteric hip fractures, and tension femoral neck stress fractures.
- Analgesics are used for pain control and are often provided parenterally.
- Muscle relaxants, antibiotics, and tetanus vaccine or booster for open fractures.
- Nursing care should focus on maintaining airway, breathing, and circulation; postoperative management of pain and infection control; assessment for hemorrhage; preparation for rehabilitation (progressive activity, lower extremity strengthening, and weight-bearing ambulation).

Joint Replacement

A total joint replacement, or arthroplasty, can be performed on any joint of the body, but knee and hip total joint replacements are the most common. More than a million are performed each year in the United States. The primary indication is disabling pain caused by severe arthritis.

Contraindications for surgery include ongoing infection or sepsis, severe vascular disease, and extensor mechanism dysfunction. The surgical goal is is pain-free joint function that enables the patient to perform activities that improve the quality of life. Complications include deep vein thrombosis, infection, periprosthetic fractures, blood loss, and nerve injury.

Where It Occurs

- Most arthroplasty procedures occur in adults older than 65 years. Both men and women have the procedure.
- Patients who have deformed joints and osteoarthritis are likely to need this procedure.
- Related factors: obesity, trauma, genetics, repetitive use, infection, rheumatoid arthritis.

Signal Symptoms

- Preoperative: pain, joint deformity, activity intolerance, altered gait, fatigue.

BE SAFE! Fractures around joint replacement prostheses are called periprosthetic fractures and are caused by surgical errors, osteoarthritis, or falls.

Diagnostic Tests

Test	What It Tells	Patient Problems/ Nursing Care
Extremity X-rays	Structure of involved bones and joints	Knowledge deficit: explain procedures.

Treatment and Nursing Care

Potential Nursing Diagnoses*

Pain (acute)
Risk for infection
Risk for injury
Activity intolerance

BE SMART! Postoperative rehabilitation is critical for the best surgical outcome.

- Postoperative monitoring occurs for 24 hours immediately after the procedure, with attention to pain relief and adequate hydration. Usually analgesia is provided through patient-controlled IV analgesia or oral analgesia.
- Early movement of the joint may occur, sometimes using a continuous passive motion (CPM) machine and exercises depending on the type of surgery.
- Most patients receive prophylactic medication treatment to prevent thromboembolism. The first outpatient visit occurs 6 weeks to 3 months after the surgery.
- Nursing care centers of pain relief, careful mobilization of the joint as prescribed, adequate hydration, thromboembolism prevention, assessing for infection, and teaching about physical activity and medications.

Limb Amputation

Amputation is the surgical severing of any body part. Amputations can be surgical (therapeutic) or traumatic (emergencies resulting from injury). The type of amputation performed in the Civil War era by a surgeon called a "sawbones" was straight across the leg, with all bone and soft tissue severed at the same level. That procedure, known as a guillotine (or open) amputation, is still seen today.

A traumatic amputation is usually the result of an industrial accident in which blades of heavy machinery sever part of a limb. A healthy young person who suffers a traumatic amputation without other injuries is often a good candidate for limb salvage. Reattachment of a limb will take place as soon as possible following the injury. The chief problems are hemorrhage and nerve damage. A closed amputation is the most common surgical procedure today. The bone is severed somewhat higher than the surrounding tissue, with a skin flap pulled over the bone end, usually from the posterior surface. This procedure provides more even pressure for a weight-bearing surface, promoting healing and more successful use of a prosthesis. In addition to severe trauma, amputations may be performed for vascular disease and tumors. It is also a wartime injury.

Where It Occurs

- In young adulthood, more men than women suffer traumatic amputations brought about by hazardous conditions in the workplace, at war, and during recreation.
- The greatest number of amputations is performed in older adults, especially men over 60, for vascular disease and tumors.

Signal Symptoms

- Postoperative: pain, infection, bleeding, gait problems, stigma.
- Postoperative: complications may include anxiety, role dysfunction, sexual dysfunction, depression.

BE SAFE! Any lacerations, abrasions, or contusions may indicate additional problems with healing and should be made known to the surgeon.

Diagnostic Tests

Test	What It Tells	Patient Problems/ Nursing Care
Ankle arm index (AAI)	Ratio of the blood pressure in the leg to that in the arm; identifies people with severe aortoiliac occlusive disease	Knowledge deficit: explain procedures.

Treatment and Nursing Care

Potential Nursing Diagnoses*

Impaired mobility
Disturbed body image
Pain (acute)
Risk for infection

BE SMART! Phantom limb pain, very real physical discomfort, usually begins about 2 weeks after surgery.

- Complete limb amputation is treated by flushing the wound with sterile normal saline, applying a sterile pressure dressing, and elevating the limb.
- Analgesics relieve pain and allow for increasing mobility to limit surgical complications.
- Wound maintenance should be the focal point of nursing care. Assess for signs of bleeding, infection, and poor wound healing.
- Rehabilitation includes not only mobility and prosthesis fitting but also medication management, emotional status, support of changing roles, prevention of infection, gait training, and balance training.

Osteoarthritis

Osteoarthritis (OA) is a degenerative disorder of the movable joints, characterized by abrasion and deterioration of the articular cartilage, with new bone formation at joint surfaces. It is classified as primary or secondary. Primary, or idiopathic, OA occurs without underlying abnormality or cause and is considered to be a normal consequence of the aging process. Secondary OA has a clearly identifiable cause, such as trauma, an underlying congenital anomaly, a metabolic disturbance such as gout or acromegaly, or inflammatory processes.

Where It Occurs

- Incidence increases with age.
- Rates appear to be lower in northern climates.

- In patients younger than 55, men and women are affected equally, but in patients older than 55, the condition is more common in women, except in the hips, where it is more common in men.
- Most common locations: weight-bearing joints, including the knees, hips, spine, and feet. Other sites: distal interphalangeal (DIP) and proximal interphalangeal (PIP) joints of the hands.

Signal Symptoms

- Joint pain; dull, aching, generalized discomfort; joint swelling.
- Activity intolerance, morning stiffness, impaired gait, decreased joint mobility, stiffness during rest (gelling).
- Weight gain, decreased physical activity.

BE SAFE! Assess the patient's gait and home environment to determine the risk for falls and fractures.

Diagnostic Tests

Test	What It Tells	Patient Problems/ Nursing Care
Erythrocyte sedimentation rate (ESR)	Normal in primary OA but high in inflammatory process	Knowledge deficit: explain procedures. Patient will need venipuncture.
Rheumatoid factor	Normal in primary OA	Knowledge deficit: explain procedures. Patient will need venipuncture.

Treatment and Nursing Care

Potential Nursing Diagnoses*

Pain (acute and chronic)
Activity intolerance
Impaired mobility
Risk for falls
Knowledge deficit (medications, lifestyle, rest and activity)

BE SMART! If patient is on corticosteroids or NSAIDs (see below) observe for GI distress and complications such as bleeding or epigastric distress.

■ Goals are to decrease stress on involved joints, maintain function, and reduce pain.
■ Analgesia is used to relieve pain; NSAIDs are used frequently in OA to relieve pain and swelling. Other drugs include corticosteroids, sodium hyaluronate, acetaminophen, muscle relaxants, calcium supplements if needed.
■ Hot and cold physical therapies are used to reduce pain, improve range of motion, and maintain patient's ability to function.
■ Surgical methods may be implemented when disease is advanced.
■ Teach patient about physical activity, medications, and how to avoid injury and exacerbations.

Osteomyelitis

Osteomyelitis is an infection of bone, bone marrow, and the soft tissue that surrounds the bone. It is generally caused by pyogenic (pus-producing) bacteria but may be the result of a viral or fungal infection. Osteomyelitis may be an acute or chronic condition. Acute osteomyelitis is an infection that is less than 1 month in duration from the time of the initial infection. Chronic osteomyelitis refers to a bone infection that persists for longer than 4 weeks or represents a persistent problem with periods of remission and exacerbations.

Osteomyelitis most commonly occurs in the long bones and, in particular, the tibia, femur, and fibula. The metaphysis (growing portion of a bone) of the distal portion of the femur and the proximal portion of the tibia are the most frequent sites because of the sluggish blood supply that occurs in those areas. After gaining entrance to the bone, the bacteria grow and form an abscess, which spreads along the shaft of the bone under the periosteum. Pressure elevates the periosteum, destroying its blood vessels and causing bone necrosis. The dead bone tissue (sequestra) cannot easily be liquefied and removed. The body's healing response is to lay new bone (involucrum) over the sequestra. However, the sequestra is a perfect environment for bacteria, and chronic osteomyelitis occurs if the bacteria are not eliminated. Primary causes are vascular insufficiency, trauma, and diabetes mellitus.

Where It Occurs

- The acute form of osteomyelitis is most frequently found in children, while the chronic form is most commonly observed in adults.
- Hematogenous osteomyelitis generally occurs in boys from the age of 1 to 12.

Signal Symptoms

- Local infectious symptoms: redness, swelling, and increased warmth; fever, malaise, fatigue, activity intolerance.
- A foul-smelling draining wound may be present, with an intense pain or tenderness over the affected bone, and muscle spasms.
- Late: problems with weight bearing, poor range of motion, deformity.

BE SAFE! Treatment of infection is the highest priority to reduce long-term complications.

Diagnostic Tests

Test	What It Tells	Patient Problems/ Nursing Care
Bone scan	Identifies areas of infection and changes in blood flow resulting from inflammation	Knowledge deficit: explain procedures.
Bone biopsy	Identifies organisms and bacterial sensitivities to antibiotics	Knowledge deficit: explain procedures.

Treatment and Nursing Care

Potential Nursing Diagnoses*

Pain (acute)
Risk for infection
Activity intolerance
Risk for injury

- The most critical factor in eliminating osteomyelitis is prevention.
- Early and adequate débridement of open fractures to remove necrotic tissue limits bacterial growth.
- Antibiotics kill bacteria and decrease spread of infection.
- Nursing care centers on managing discomfort and pain, administering antibiotics, and managing wound care.

Pelvic Fracture

A pelvic fracture is a break in the integrity of either the innominate bones or the sacrum. The innominate bones are connected posteriorly at the level of the sacrum and anteriorly to the symphysis pubis. These structures form a ring of bones with ligaments that are designed to accommodate weight distributed from the trunk to the pelvis across both the sacrum and the joints at the S1 vertebra. The S1 joints are maintained by the anterior and posterior ligaments and pelvic floor ligaments. The iliac vascular structures, lumbosacral plexus, lower genitourinary tract, reproductive organs, portions of the small bowel, distal colon and rectum, iliofemoral vessels, and lumbosacral plexus bilaterally all may be affected by a pelvic fracture.

Two out of three occurrences of pelvic fractures are associated with motor vehicle crashes (MVCs) and automobile–pedestrian trauma.

Where It Occurs

- Complex pelvic fractures are more common in men and women younger than 35 years and are less frequent in patients older than 65 years.
- The overall incidence of pelvic fractures is similar for men and women, with an increase in incidence in women older than 85, perhaps because of their increased incidence of osteoporosis.
- During young adulthood, more males than females have pelvic fractures due to injuries such as MVCs.

Signal Symptoms

- Pain; misalignment of legs; accompanying scrotal, labial, flank, and inguinal hematomas; rectal and vaginal lacerations; abrasions, ecchymosis, or contusions over bony prominences, the groin, genitalia, and suprapubic area; blood at urethral opening.
- Internal rotation of the lower extremity, or "frog leg positioning," is suggestive of pelvic ring abnormalities.
- Accompanying spinal injuries.

BE SAFE! In people with pelvic fractures, ecchymosis or hematoma formation over the pubis or blood at the urinary meatus is significant for associated lower genitourinary tract trauma.

Diagnostic Tests

Test	What It Tells	Patient Problems/ Nursing Care
Pelvic x-rays	Demonstrates radiographic evidence of pelvic injury	Knowledge deficit: explain procedures.
Ultrasound; focused assessment with sonography for trauma	Shows location of bleeding to explain shock	Knowledge deficit: explain procedures.

Treatment and Nursing Care

Potential Nursing Diagnoses*

Fluid volume deficit
Pain (acute)
Risk for injury
Mobility, bed, impaired
Knowledge deficit (medications, pain relief, mobility)

BE SMART! Retroperitoneal hemorrhage is a serious complication that may be masked by other symptoms. Assess for fluid volume deficit (tachycardia, delayed capillary blanching, decreased urinary output).

- Bedrest alone can manage some fractures.
- Internal fixation restores the pelvis to its original anatomic configuration.
- Narcotic analgesics provide pain relief.
- Maintenance of airway, breathing, and circulation, along with wound care, are the highest priorities for nursing care.
- Patient will need rehabilitation and postoperative instruction.

Polymyalgia Rheumatica

Polymyalgia rheumatica (PMR) is a condition characterized by pain, often in the hip and shoulder. Many patients suffer from stiffness in the morning that can be lengthy in duration. The cause of the condition is unknown, but PMR is likely of genetic origin with contributing environmental factors.

Where It Occurs

- The condition is almost exclusively found in Northern European whites but is sometimes found in African Americans.
- Females are twice as likely as males to suffer from PMR.
- Incidence increases with age; PMR is typically found in patients older than 50.

Signal Symptoms

- Pain often localizes in upper arms, neck, and shoulders. Pain occurs without swelling but is associated with bilateral myalgia, morning stiffness, decreased range of motion.
- Low-grade fever, fatigue, weight loss, depression.
- Late: muscle atrophy, carpal tunnel syndrome, giant cell arteritis with visual changes.

BE SAFE! Protect the patient from falls and further injury to joints, bones, and soft tissues. This is especially true if the patient has visual changes.

Test	What It Tells	Patient Problems/ Nursing Care
Erythrocyte sedimentation rate (ESR)	Rate is elevated	Knowledge deficit: explain procedures. Patient will need venipuncture.
C-reactive protein levels	Levels are elevated	Knowledge deficit: explain procedures. Patient will need venipuncture.

Treatment and Nursing Care

Potential Nursing Diagnoses*

Pain (acute and chronic)
Activity intolerance
Impaired mobility
Risk for falls
Knowledge deficit (medications, lifestyle, rest and activity)

BE SMART! Teach patient how to manage exacerbations, physical activity, and lifestyle.

- Corticosteroids can be administered to alleviate symptoms.
- NSAIDs can be prescribed in mild cases.
- Methotrexate, azathioprine, and other immunosuppressive drugs may be used.
- Occupational and physical therapy might be helpful to maintain function.
- Surgical methods may be implemented when disease is advanced for giant cell arteritis.
- Teach patient about physical activity, medications, and how to avoid injury and exacerbations.

Shoulder Dislocation

A shoulder dislocation is displacement, separation, or malalignment of the scapula and humerus. Dislocations commonly occur anteriorly at the lower front of the shoulder but also occur posteriorly, inferiorly, or anterior-superiorly. Once a shoulder dislocation occurs, patients are prone to redislocation (repeat dislocations). Subluxation refers to a partial dislocation; a dislocation is a 100% subluxation.

When dislocation or subluxation is caused by trauma, associated injuries generally occur to the blood vessels, nerves, ligaments, and soft tissues that surround the joint. In addition to the damage at the joint, tissue death from circulatory compromise to the distal extremity or permanent nerve damage from edema can occur. Avascular necrosis (death of bone cells because of inadequate blood supply) may occur if the bone is torn away from its normal position next to the vascular-rich bony surface.

Where It Occurs

■ Traumatic dislocations occur most frequently in persons under 20 years of age as a result of their involvement in sports or risk-taking activities.
■ In general, more men than women are injured in violent events.

Signal Symptoms

■ At the time of injury, a sense of "popping" and numbness running down the length of the arm.
■ Severe pain, inability to move the extremity, a change in the length of the extremities, abnormal contour of the joint, and ecchymosis (bruising).

BE SAFE! Make sure to remove all of the patient's clothing to observe skin surfaces.

Diagnostic Tests

Test	What It Tells	Patient Problems/ Nursing Care
Radiological examination	Assessment of dislocations should include two views (90 degrees to each other, and of affected area with joints above and below)	Knowledge deficit: explain all procedures. Medicate for pain.

Potential Nursing Diagnoses*

Pain (acute)
Impaired physical mobility
Risk for injury
Risk for infection (if surgery is needed)
Knowledge deficit (prevention of redislocation, medications, alignment)

BE SMART! This injury is extremely painful. Pain control is the first priority.

■ The primary goal for therapeutic management is to realign the bones of the joint to their normal anatomic position.
■ NSAIDs may inhibit cyclooxygenase activity and prostaglandin synthesis.
■ Analgesics and sedatives are used to achieve easily arousable analgesia and sedation so that ongoing assessments can occur.
■ Nursing care focuses on pain relief, maintaining proper arm and shoulder alignment, and prevention of further injury.

Bell's Palsy

Bell's palsy is characterized by acute, unilateral facial muscle weakness or paralysis as the result of cranial nerve VII (facial nerve) inflammation and swelling of the nerve within the facial canal. The condition may be caused by a virus, such as herpes simplex type I or HIV, or a bacteria, such as syphilis or Lyme disease. The condition affects up to 40,000 people each year in the United States.

Where It Occurs

- Bell's palsy is more common in individuals over the age of 30.
- Genetics may play a role.
- People with diabetes mellitus may be more affected than the general population.

Signal Symptoms

- Facial paralysis or weakness, mild numbness on the affected side, and visible sagging in the face are all possible symptoms.
- Symptoms are usually unilateral.
- Early symptoms may resemble a viral infection; facial weakness follows in 2 to 3 days.

BE SAFE! Monitor the patient's ability to eat and swallow so that the airway is not compromised.

Diagnostic Tests

Test	What It Tells	Patient Problems/ Nursing Care
Computerized tomography scan	Rules out masses, tumors, or growths	Knowledge deficit: explain all procedures.

Treatment and Nursing Care

Potential Nursing Diagnoses*

Ineffective airway clearance
Coping (individual)
Anxiety
Risk for compromised human dignity

BE SMART! If the patient cannot close the eye, eye drops or an eye patch at night may help keep the surface of the eye moist.

- Steroids such as methylprednisolone reduce inflammation and edema; may reduce long-term symptoms.
- Analgesics manage pain.
- Physical therapy may be appropriate.
- Provide support and counseling because of changes in appearance and concern over long-term consequences.

Cancer, Brain

Primary brain tumors develop from various tissue types within the intracranial cavity and are named for the tissue in which they originate (e.g., astrocytomas originate in the astrocytes). Tumors are customarily described as benign or malignant; however, all brain tumors may be considered malignant because without treatment, the patient dies. Even well-contained tumors may lead to serious consequences because they compress or invade neighboring structures within the enclosed skull. Brain tumors cause their symptoms directly by destroying neurons or indirectly by exerting pressure, displacing brain structures, and increasing intracranial pressure (ICP). Besides primary tumors arising from intracranial tissue, metastatic tumors may also migrate to the area by hematogenous spread. Common sources for brain metastases are the lung, breast, and colon.

Types of brain tumors include glioblastoma multiform (spongioblastoma), astrocytoma, medulloblastoma, ependymoma, oligodendroglioma, meningioma, schwannoma (acoustic neurinoma, neurilemma), pituitary adenoma, and lymphoma.

Where It Occurs

■ African Americans, especially African American women, have a slightly higher incidence of meningiomas and pituitary adenomas.
■ Most central nervous system (CNS) tumors occur in patients over 45, with the peak incidence found after age 70.

Signal Symptoms

■ Headache, dizziness, progressive neurological deficit, convulsions (focal or generalized), increased ICP, and organic mental changes.
■ Structural abnormalities depending on the type and location of the tumor may be present.

BE SAFE! Protect the patient from falls by surveying the environment, assessing patient's decision-making ability, and providing mobility assistance when needed.

Diagnostic Tests

Test	What It Tells	Patient Problems/ Nursing Care
Computed tomography and magnetic resonance imaging	Locates size, location, and extent of tumor	Knowledge deficit: explain procedures.

Treatment and Nursing Care

Potential Nursing Diagnoses*

Decreased intracranial adaptive capacity
Ineffective airway clearance
Pain (acute)
Disturbed body image
Risk for falls
Impaired memory

> **BE SMART!** Patient education is critical following all treatment options.

- The type of treatment used for brain cancer depends on the type of tumor, but primary modes of treatment include surgery, radiotherapy, and pharmacologic therapy.
- Chemotherapy plays a very minor role in treatment of brain metastases because the blood–brain barrier prevents delivery to the tumor of the cytotoxic agents in high concentrations.
- Nursing care focuses on managing the airway and maximizing patient comfort.

Cerebral Aneurysm

Cerebral aneurysm is an outpouching of the wall of a cerebral artery that results from weakening of the wall of the vessel. Cerebral aneurysms have a variety of sizes, shapes, and causes. Aneurysms can be small, large, giant, or supergiant in size; berry, saccular, or fusiform in shape; and traumatic, Charcot-Bouchard, or dissecting in etiology. Most cerebral aneurysms are saccular or berrylike with a stem and a neck.

Clinical concern arises if an aneurysm ruptures or becomes large enough to exert pressure on surrounding structures. When the vessel wall becomes so thin that it can no longer withstand the surrounding arterial pressure, the cerebral aneurysm ruptures, causing direct hemorrhaging of arterial blood into the subarachnoid space (*subarachnoid hemorrhage*).

Where It Occurs

- The peak incidence of cerebral aneurysm occurs between 35 and 60 years of age.
- Women in their late 40s through mid-50s are affected slightly more than men.
- The odds of African Americans having a cerebral aneurysm are approximately twice that of whites.
- Causes are likely to be multifactorial and are a combination of environmental factors, such as hypertension, and a genetic predisposition.

Signal Symptoms

■ Before rupture, cerebral aneurysms are usually asymptomatic but oculomotor nerve (cranial nerve III) palsy may occur.
■ Headache, facial pain, alterations in consciousness, seizures, blurred vision.
■ Stiff neck, back or leg pain, or photophobia, as well as hearing noises or throbbing (bruits) in the head.

BE SAFE! About 10% of people with aneurysmal subarachnoid hemorrhage die before reaching the hospital. Early surgical intervention is essential.

Diagnostic Tests

Test	What It Tells	Patient Problems/ Nursing Care
Cerebral angiogram	Radiographic views of cerebral circulation show interruptions to circulation or changes in vessel wall appearance	Knowledge deficit: explain procedures. Check for allergies to contrast media and monitor mental status.
Computed tomography	Shows anterior to posterior slices of the brain to highlight abnormalities	Knowledge deficit: explain procedures.

Treatment and Nursing Care

Potential Nursing Diagnoses*

Ineffective tissue perfusion (cerebral)
Pain (acute)
Disturbed body image
Risk for confusion (acute)

- The first priority is to evaluate and support airway, breathing, and circulation.
- Surgery is indicated to prevent rupture or rebleeding of the cerebral artery.
- Calcium channel blockers prevent vasospasm and hypertension.
- Corticosteroids reduce swelling.
- If surgery is performed, postoperative nursing care includes venous draining.

Cerebral Concussion

Cerebral concussion is a transient, temporary, neurogenic dysfunction caused by mechanical force to the brain. Cerebral concussions are the most common form of head injury. Concussions are classified as mild or classic on the basis of the degree of symptoms, particularly those of unconsciousness and memory loss. Mild concussion is a temporary neurological dysfunction without loss of consciousness or memory. Classic concussion includes temporary neurological dysfunction with unconsciousness and memory loss. Recovery from concussion usually takes minutes to hours. Most concussion patients recover fully within 48 hours, but subtle residual impairment may occur. The most widely accepted theory for concussion is that acceleration–deceleration forces cause the injury.

In rare cases, a secondary injury caused by cerebral hypoxia and ischemia can lead to cerebral edema and increased intracranial pressure (ICP). Some patients develop a postconcussion syndrome (postinjury sequelae after a mild head injury). Symptoms may be experienced for several weeks and, in unusual circumstances, may last up to 1 year. In rare situations, patients who experience multiple concussions may suffer long-term brain damage. Complications of cerebral concussion include seizures or persistent vomiting. In rare instances, a concussion may lead to intracranial hemorrhage (subdural, parenchymal, or epidural).

Where It Occurs

- Males are affected at higher rates than are females.
- Most instances of cerebral concussion occur in the first four decades of life.
- Most common causes are motor vehicle collisions, sports-related injuries, and alcohol- and/or drug-related trauma.

Signal Symptoms

- Transient confusion, possible loss of consciousness, momentary loss of reflexes, arrest of respirations, possible retrograde or anterograde amnesia.
- Headache, drowsiness, dizziness, irritability, giddiness, visual disturbances (seeing stars), and gait disturbances.

BE SAFE! People with changes in mental status and loss of consciousness need to be assessed by a health-care provider.

Diagnostic Tests

Test	What It Tells	Patient Problems/ Nursing Care
Computed tomography	Identification of size and location of site of injury	Knowledge deficit: explain all procedures.

Treatment and Nursing Care

Potential Nursing Diagnoses*

Disturbed thought processes
Pain (acute)
Ineffective tissue perfusion (cerebral)
Risk for injury

BE SMART! Assess the patient's mental status frequently with pupil checks after the acute phase of injury.

- Treatment generally consists of bedrest with the head of the bed elevated at least 30 degrees, observation, and pain relief.
- Acetaminophen manages headache.
- For patients with serious head injury, ICP monitoring may be necessary.
- Nursing care includes educating the patient and his or her significant others about medications and possible complications.
- Knowledge deficit (physical activity, medications, rehabilitation).

Encephalitis

Encephalitis, or inflammation of the brain, usually occurs when the cerebral hemispheres, brainstem, or cerebellum is infected by a micro-organism. Encephalitis has two forms: primary and postinfectious (or parainfectious). Although fungi and autoimmune disorders can cause encephalitis, the primary form of the disease occurs when a virus invades and replicates within the brain. Postinfectious encephalitis describes brain inflammation that develops in combination with other viral illnesses or following the administration of vaccines such as measles, mumps, and rubella. In that case, encephalitis occurs because of a hypersensitivity reaction that leads to demyelination of nerves.

When the brain becomes inflamed, lymphocytes infiltrate brain tissue and the meninges of the brain. Cerebral edema results, and ultimately, brain cells can degenerate, leading to widespread nerve cell destruction.

Where It Occurs

- Encephalitis caused by herpes simplex virus (HSV) type 1 is most common in children and young adults.
- La Crosse encephalitis is most common in children from 5 to 10 years of age.
- Eastern equine encephalitis (EEE) commonly occurs in children younger than 10 and in older adults, whereas western equine encephalitis (WEE) occurs in infants under a year and in older adults.
- St. Louis encephalitis is seen most often in adults older than 35.

Signal Symptoms

- Headache, nausea/vomiting, pupil irregularity and dilation, seizures, focal neurological deficits such as aphasia, weakness, paresthesias, hemiparesis, and decerebrate posturing (extension).
- Neurological signs and symptoms depend on the location, rapidity, and source of bleeding.

BE SAFE! Note that approximately one-third of patients with an epidural hematoma have initial unconsciousness followed by a period of lucidity and then subsequent unconsciousness. Make sure patients with loss of consciousness have a complete workup.

Diagnostic Tests

Test	What It Tells	Patient Problems/ Nursing Care
Computed tomography scan	Visualizes structural abnormalities, including skull fractures, soft tissue abnormalities, hemorrhage, cerebral edema, and shifting brain structures	Knowledge deficit: explain procedures.
Radiological examination: skull, chest and cervical (all cervical vertebrae including C7–T1 junction) spine x-rays with anteroposterior, lateral, and open-mouth view	Determines presence of accompanying structural abnormalities	Knowledge deficit: explain procedures.

Treatment and Nursing Care

Potential Nursing Diagnoses*

Ineffective airway clearance
Pain (acute)
Confusion (acute)

Ineffective breathing pattern
Risk for injury

BE SMART! Monitor the patient's neurological status frequently with an assessment tool like the Glasgow Coma Scale.

- Endotracheal intubation and mechanical ventilation may be necessary to ensure oxygenation and ventilation and to decrease the risk of pulmonary aspiration.
- Surgical evaluation of the clot, control of the hemorrhage, and resection of nonviable brain tissue may be warranted as soon as possible.
- Sedatives, analgesics, anesthetics control intermittent increases in ICP with a resultant decrease in cerebral perfusion pressure.
- Chemical paralytic agents provide muscle relaxation needed to improve oxygenation and ventilation.
- The highest nursing priority is maintaining a patent airway, appropriate ventilation and oxygenation, and adequate circulation.

Guillain-Barré Syndrome

Guillain-Barré syndrome (GBS; also known as *acute idiopathic demyelinating polyneuropathy*) is an acute, rapidly progressing form of polyneuritis that results in a temporary, flaccid paralysis lasting for 4 to 8 weeks. Motor, sensory, and autonomic functions may be involved. The syndrome is characterized by a diffuse inflammation or demyelination (or both) of the ascending or descending peripheral nerves that leads to a viral illness and then paralysis.

The exact cause of GBS is unknown, and it seems to be a collection of clinical syndromes that present as an acute inflammatory polyradiculoneuropathy with resultant weakness and diminished reflexes. Two-thirds of patients who develop it have had a viral or bacterial infection 1 to 3 weeks before the development of symptoms.

Where It Occurs

- Most commonly, GBS affects young and middle-aged adults 30 to 50 years of age and men slightly more than women.
- Patients older than 65 have a significantly higher mortality rate than their younger counterparts.

- There are no known racial and ethnic considerations except that Asian Americans are most likely to have GBS after an infection with *Campylobacter jejuni* as compared with other agents.
- Patients often describe a recent minor upper respiratory or gastrointestinal febrile illness.

Signal Symptoms

- Patients complain of paresthesia (numbness, prickling, tingling) early in the course of the illness.
- Major neurological sign: muscle weakness; sensory loss, particularly in the legs and later in the arms, occurs as well.
- Cranial nerve involvement: facial droop, diplopia, dysarthria, dysphagia.

> **BE SAFE!** Impairment of respiratory functions, the most life-threatening effect of GBS, does not occur until the paralysis has affected all of the peripheral areas and the trunk.

Diagnostic Tests

Test	What It Tells	Patient Problems/ Nursing Care
Cerebrospinal fluid (CSF) assay	Increase in CSF protein without an increase in cell count is often noted.	Knowledge deficit: explain procedures. Remain with patient to reduce anxiety, and position the patient properly.

Treatment and Nursing Care

Potential Nursing Diagnoses*

Ineffective airway clearance
Activity intolerance
Risk for neurovascular dysfunction
Impaired physical mobility
Anxiety

- The most important interventions center on maintaining a patent airway and adequate breathing.
- During the acute phase of the illness, the patient may be in the intensive care unit, particularly to support pulmonary function with endotracheal intubation and mechanical ventilation.
- Antihypertensives control hypertensive episodes.
- Heparin prevents thromboembolism during periods of immobility.
- Nursing care involves supportive management of the neurological and cardiopulmonary systems, reducing anxiety, explaining procedures and prognosis, and planning for rehabilitation.

Headache—Cluster and Migraine

Migraine headache is a primary headache syndrome that is an episodic vascular disorder with or without a common aura. A migraine headache is a prototype of a vascular headache, which involves vasodilation and localized inflammation. Ultimately, arteries are sensitized to pain. Cerebral blood flow is diminished before the onset of the headache and is increased during the actual episode. Most migraine sufferers have a trigger, or precipitating factor, associated with the onset of symptoms.

Migraine headaches are of two types: classic migraine and common migraine. Classic migraine has a prodromal (preheadache) phase that lasts approximately 15 minutes and is accompanied by disturbances of neurological functioning such as visual disturbances, speech disturbances, and paresthesias. Neurological symptoms cease with the beginning of the headache, which is often accompanied by nausea and vomiting. Common migraine does not have a preheadache phase but is characterized by an immediate onset of a throbbing headache. Although the causes of migraine headache are uncertain, a commonly held theory is that early vasoconstriction and subsequent vasodilation occur because of the release of biologically active amines such as serotonin, dopamine, norepinephrine, and epinephrine.

Where It Occurs

- Begins in childhood or puberty; affects females more than males; continues sporadically until middle age but uncommon during the elder years.
- Migraine headaches have a higher prevalence among whites than among African Americans and Asian Americans.
- Hormonal changes associated with pregnancy, menstruation, and menopause may trigger migraines.

Signal Symptoms

- Common migraines have an immediate onset of unilateral throbbing pain and nausea.
- Transient visual, motor, sensory, cognitive, or psychic disturbance that lasts up to 15 minutes and precedes the headache.
- Scotomas, photophobia, or visual scintillations.

BE SAFE! The main goal is to stop or prevent progression of the symptoms or reverse a headache that has begun.

Diagnostic Tests

No test is diagnostic for migraine headaches. The following tests may be necessary for differential diagnosis: computed tomography scan, skull x-ray, cranial nerve testing, arteriogram, lumbar puncture, cerebrospinal fluid testing, electroencephalogram, and magnetic resonance imaging.

Treatment and Nursing Care

Potential Nursing Diagnoses*

Pain (acute)
Nausea
Anxiety
Knowledge deficit (medications)

BE SMART! Teach patients to avoid certain foods that may be triggers: alcohol, caffeine, chocolates, aspartame, saccharin, monosodium glutamate (MSG), citrus fruits, and meats with nitrites.

- Nonnarcotic analgesics abort or relieve a migraine headache.
- Prochlorperazine also relieves a migraine headache.
- Medications used to relieve pain: selective serotonin receptor (5-HT1) agonists (triptans), ergot alkaloids, NSAIDs. Prophylactic medications: antiepileptic drugs, beta blockers, tricyclic antidepressants, calcium channel blockers.
- Nurses should teach the patient to avoid triggers that may lead to headaches: stress, change in sleep patterns, cigarette smoking, exposure to fluorescent lighting, infections, fatigue, ingestion of ice.

Meningitis

Meningitis is an acute or subacute inflammation of the meninges (lining of the brain and spinal cord). The bacterial or viral pathogens responsible for meningitis usually come from another site, such as those that lead to an upper respiratory infection, sinusitis, or mumps. The organisms can also enter the meninges through open wounds. Bacterial meningitis is considered a medical emergency because the outcome depends on the interval between the onset of disease and the initiation of antimicrobial therapy. In contrast, the viral form of meningitis is sometimes called *aseptic* or *serous* meningitis. It is usually self-limiting and, in contrast to the bacterial form, is often described as benign.

In the bacterial form, bacteria enter the meningeal space and elicit an inflammatory response. This process includes the release of a purulent exudate that is spread to other areas of the brain by the cerebrospinal fluid (CSF). If the infection invades the brain tissue, the disease is then classified as encephalitis.

Where It Occurs

- Meningitis occurs most frequently in young children, elderly people, and persons in a debilitated state.
- Infants and the very old are at the most risk for pneumococcal meningitis, whereas children from 2 months to 3 years most frequently have hemophilus meningitis.
- In the United States, African Americans are at greater risk than other races and ethnicities, although at this time there is no explanation for those differences in risk.

Signal Symptoms

- Subacute: mild symptoms such as irritability, loss of appetite, and headaches.
- Acute: headache that becomes progressively worse, with accompanying vomiting, disorientation, delirium, photophobia.
- Nuchal rigidity or discomfort on neck flexion, Kernig sign (inability to extend legs when lying supine), Brudzinski sign (flexion of hips when neck is flexed from supine position), nausea, vomiting, pupil changes.

BE SAFE! If mental status deteriorates, make sure patient has an open airway and adequate breathing.

Diagnostic Tests

Test	What It Tells	Patient Problems/ Nursing Care
Head computed tomography scan with contrast or magnetic resonance imaging with gadolinium	Increased intracranial pressure (ICP) may result from infection and lead to intracranial changes	Knowledge deficit: explain procedures.
Lumbar puncture for CSF analysis	Identifies invading microorganisms	Knowledge deficit: explain procedures. Postprocedure pain. Risk for infection at site of puncture.

Treatment and Nursing Care

Potential Nursing Diagnoses*

Risk for infection
Ineffective airway clearance
Impaired mobility
Risk for aspiration
Confusion (acute)

- The most critical treatment is the rapid initiation of antibiotic therapy, which causes bacterial lysis and prevents continuation of infection.
- In addition, assessment and maintenance of airway, breathing, and circulation (ABCs) are essential.
- Other strategies to manage increased ICP include osmotic diuretics, such as mannitol, or intraventricular CSF drainage and ICP pressure monitoring.
- In the acute phase, the primary nursing goals are to preserve neurological function and to provide comfort. In the recovery phase, the patient may need rehabilitation and also education about medications, physical activity, nutrition, and lifestyle.

Multiple Sclerosis

Multiple sclerosis (MS) is a chronic, progressive degenerative disease that affects the myelin sheath of the white matter of the brain and spinal cord. The disease affects quality rather than duration of life. In MS, nerve impulses are conducted between the brain and the spinal cord along neurons protected by the myelin sheath, which is a highly conductive fatty material. When plaques form on the myelin sheath, causing inflammation and eventual demyelination, nerve transmission becomes erratic. Areas commonly involved are the optic nerves, cerebrum, and cervical spinal cord.

Four forms of MS have been identified. Benign MS, which affects approximately 20% of patients, causes mild disability; infrequent, mild, early attacks are followed by almost complete recovery. Exacerbating-remitting MS, which affects approximately 25% of patients, is marked by frequent attacks that start early in the course of the illness, followed by less complete clearing of signs and symptoms than in benign MS. Chronic relapsing MS, which affects approximately 40% of patients, has fewer, less complete remissions after an exacerbation than has exacerbating-remitting MS. Chronic relapsing MS has a cumulative progression, with more symptoms occurring during each new attack. The fourth form of MS, chronic progressive, afflicts approximately 15% of patients and is similar to chronic relapsing MS except that the onset is more subtle and the disease progresses slowly without remission. The cause of MS is unknown.

Where It Occurs

■ MS is more prevalent in colder climates, in urban areas, and among whites.
■ MS affects women more than men with a 2:1 ratio.
■ Roughly 70% of patients experience the onset of MS between the ages of 20 and 40, while 20% of patients experience the onset of the disease between the ages of 40 and 60.

Signal Symptoms

■ Vague and unrelated symptoms; involuntary, rhythmic movements of the eyes (nystagmus).
■ Sensory loss of the trunk and limbs, muscle cramping, bladder dysfunction, bowel dysfunction, sexual dysfunction.
■ Dizziness, fatigue, insomnia, pain, short attention span, depression, euphoria.

BE SAFE! Teach the patient to reduce stress and decrease fatigue levels, which will likely improve symptoms.

Diagnostic Tests

Test	What It Tells	Patient Problems/ Nursing Care
Cerebrospinal fluid (CSF) analysis	Elevated protein level (increased WBCs) reflects immune response	Knowledge deficit: explain procedures. Patient positioning. Remain with patient to reduce anxiety.

Treatment and Nursing Care

Potential Nursing Diagnoses*

Impaired physical mobility
Ineffective role performance
Disturbed sensory perception, kinesthetic

Anxiety

Knowledge deficit (physical activity, stress reduction, medications)

> **BE SMART!** MS is a chronic disease that requires lifestyle changes and risk reduction. Make sure the patient has a social service consultation and support to make decisions about treatment choices.

- Most medical treatment is designed to slow disease progression and address the symptoms, such as urinary retention, spasticity, and motor and speech deficits.
- Corticosteroids help decrease symptoms and induce remissions through anti-inflammatory effects.
- Immunomodulatory agents help decrease symptoms and induce remissions.
- Nursing care centers on instructing the patient how to manage symptoms and changes in lifestyle.

Myasthenia Gravis

Myasthenia gravis (MG) is an autoimmune disease that produces fatigue and voluntary muscle weakness, both of which become worse with exercise and improve with rest. The muscles that are frequently involved include those for eye and eyelid movement, chewing and swallowing, breathing, and movement of the distal muscles of the extremities. This weakness progressively worsens during the day or at times of stress, so the greatest fatigue is likely to occur at the end of the day. MG frequently accompanies disorders of the immune system or the thyroid gland.

Rapid acute exacerbations are classified as either myasthenic or cholinergic crises. Both crises lead to extreme respiratory distress, difficulty in swallowing and speaking, great anxiety, and generalized weakness, thus making differentiation challenging but crucial for selection of appropriate intensive therapy. Myasthenic crisis is caused by under-medication, whereas a cholinergic crisis results from excessive anticho-linesterase medication and is likely to occur within 45 to 60 minutes of the last drug dosage.

Where It Occurs

- In people in the age range of 20 to 30 years, women are more often affected than men; in the later years (over 50 years old), men are more likely than women to be affected.
- Neonatal MG occurs in 10% to 20% of infants with myasthenic mothers.

Signal Symptoms

- Changes that involve the eyes, such as ptosis (eyelid drooping), diplopia (double vision), reduced eye closure, and blurred vision, are often the earliest signs of MG.
- A masklike or "snarling" appearance may be visible because of the involvement of the facial muscles.
- Muscle and limb weakness, dysphagia, weakness of head and neck flexion.

BE SAFE! The inability to maintain an open airway and adequate breathing is life threatening.

Diagnostic Tests

Test	What It Tells	Patient Problems/ Nursing Care
Anti-acetylcholine receptor (AChR) antibody	Positive result for anti-AChR antibody (Ab) is found in 74% of patients (80% of patients with generalized myasthenia and 50% of those with ocular myasthenia)	Knowledge deficit: explain procedures. Patient will need venipuncture.
AChR antibody test	Detects presence of antibodies against the AChR in serum	Knowledge deficit: explain procedures. Patient will need venipuncture.

Treatment and Nursing Care

Potential Nursing Diagnoses*

Ineffective airway clearance
Ineffective breathing pattern
Activity intolerance
Fatigue
Ineffective coping
Knowledge deficit

BE SMART! As the disease progresses, have the patient and family speak with palliative care health professionals.

- There is no cure for MG; treatment is predominantly pharmacologic.
- Anticholinesterase drugs block the action of the enzyme anticholinesterase, thereby producing symptomatic improvement.
- Prednisone suppresses the autoimmune activity of MG.
- The primary acute nursing concerns focus on the adequacy of the patient's airway and breathing. Long-term considerations include home health care, home ventilator management, and palliative care.

Parkinson's Disease

Parkinson's disease (PD) is a clinical condition characterized by gradual slowing of voluntary movement (bradykinesia); muscular rigidity; stooped posture; distinctive gait with short, accelerating steps; diminished facial expression; and resting tremor. The disease occurs with progressive parkinsonism in the absence of a toxic or known etiology and is a progressively degenerative disease of the substantia nigra and basal ganglia. PD is also called *paralysis agitans*.

PD is caused by a degeneration of the substantia nigra in the basal ganglia of the midbrain, which leads to depletion of the neurotransmitter dopamine (DA). DA is normally produced and stored in this location and promotes smooth, purposeful movements and modulation of motor function. Depletion of DA leads to impairment of the extrapyramidal tracts and consequent loss of movement coordination. Almost 80% of DA neurons are lost before the patient begins to have the motor signs of PD. The cause is unknown.

Where It Occurs

- The average patient age is 60 years.
- PD affects men slightly more often than it does women.
- Hispanics/Latinos and whites have a higher incidence of PD than do African Americans.

Signal Symptoms

- Three cardinal signs of PD are involuntary tremors, akinesia, and progressive muscle rigidity.
- First symptom of PD is a coarse resting tremor of the fingers and thumb (pill-rolling movement) of one hand.
- Rigidity, gait difficulty, decreased dexterity, shuffling gait.

BE SAFE! Patients with PD are at risk for falls and injury. Assess gait and home environment, and make changes to prevent falls.

Diagnostic Tests

Test	What It Tells	Patient Problems/ Nursing Care
Positron emission tomography and single-photon emission computed tomography	Degeneration of substantia nigra in the basal ganglia of midbrain leads to depletion of DA	Knowledge deficit: explain procedures.

Treatment and Nursing Care

Potential Nursing Diagnoses*

Self-care deficit
Activity intolerance
Fatigue
Risk for injury
Deficient diversional activity

- To control tremor and rigidity, pharmacologic management is the treatment of choice.
- Antiparkinson drugs control tremor and rigidity.
- Amantadine hydrochloride (Symmetrel) controls tremor and rigidity by increasing the release of DA to the basal ganglia.
- Nursing care centers on helping patient adjust to life with PD and promoting independence in the patient's daily activities.

Seizure Disorder

Seizure disorder, or epilepsy, is a paroxysmal neurological disorder characterized by recurrent episodes of convulsive movements or other motor activity, loss of consciousness, sensory disturbances, and other behavioral abnormalities. Because epilepsy occurs in more than 50 diseases, it is considered a syndrome rather than a disease. The current classification for seizures was redefined in the 1980s. The characteristics of seizures depend on the focus or location of brain involvement. Seizures can vary from almost imperceptible alterations in the level of consciousness to a sudden loss of consciousness with tonic-clonic convulsions of all extremities accompanied by urinal and fecal incontinence and amnesia for the event.

Status epilepticus is more than 30 minutes of unconsciousness with continuous or intermittent convulsive seizure activity. Usually, status epilepticus results when more than six seizures occur in 24 hours or when the patient progresses from one seizure to the next without resolution of the postictal period. *Pseudoseizures* are the physical appearance of seizure activity without the cerebral electrical activity. Seizures may be caused by primary central nervous system (CNS), metabolic, or systemic disorders, or they may be idiopathic.

Where It Occurs

- Although epilepsy can occur in any age group, usually the onset is before the age of 20.
- Epilepsy occurs in all races and ethnicities, and it affects males and females equally.

Signal Symptoms

- Seizures vary greatly. Think about the following when trying to describe the seizure: Was the seizure preceded by any warning or aura? What did the patient do during the seizure? Does the patient have any recollection of the seizure? How did the patient feel after the seizure? How long did it last? How often do they occur?
- Simple partial-onset seizures: aura warning of the seizure, preserved consciousness, lasts a few seconds to a few minutes.
- Complex partial-onset seizures: impaired consciousness, behavioral arrest, staring, automatisms (chewing, mumbling, lip smacking, fumbling with hands) and lasting 60 to 90 seconds followed by postictal confusion.
- Absence seizures: brief, 20-second seizures, impaired consciousness with no aura or postictal confusion.
- Myoclonic seizures: brief, 1-second arrhythmic, jerking, motor movements.
- Clonic seizures: rhythmic, jerking motor movements with or without impairment of consciousness.
- Tonic seizures: sudden (2-5 seconds) tonic extension or flexion of the head, trunk, or extremities.
- Grand mal seizures (tonic-clonic): sudden (2–5 seconds) tonic extension of extremities followed by clonic rhythmic movements. Patients have postictal confusion. No aura.

BE SAFE! Make sure patient has an open airway and adequate breathing. Don't force anything into the mouth if the teeth are clenched during the seizure.

Diagnostic Tests

Test	What It Tells	Patient Problems/ Nursing Care
Magnetic resonance imaging	Assesses the CNS for changes in brain structure such as atrophy of certain areas or brain tumors	Knowledge deficit: explain all procedures.
Electroencephalogram	Records electrical potentials based on distribution of waveforms generated by cerebral cortex of brain; waveforms demonstrate abnormal patterns during seizures	Knowledge deficit: explain all procedures.

Treatment and Nursing Care

Potential Nursing Diagnoses*

Ineffective airway clearance
Ineffective breathing pattern
Risk for injury
Disturbed body image
Impaired memory

BE SMART! Because the patient may bite his or her tongue during the seizure, assess the patient for mouth and tongue injury.

- In general, the management of seizures is done pharmacologically.
- Surgical management may be utilized in cases of intractable epilepsy.
- Anticonvulsants such as lorazepam (Ativan) or diazepam (Valium) may be used to stop seizures quickly; other drugs are used depending on the classification.
- The most important nursing interventions are to maintain adequate airway, breathing, and circulation during the seizure and to prevent injury. Patient and family need teaching on seizure management. Activity restrictions on driving vehicles, swimming and water sports, use of power tools, and cooking with open flame are likely necessary. Counseling may be needed to manage lifestyle changes.

Spinal Cord Injury

Spinal cord injury (SCI) is trauma to the spinal cord, with half of the injuries producing paraplegia and half quadriplegia. A physiological cascade of events occurs at the time of an SCI and leads to neuronal damage and neurological deficit. The initial injury causes a release of glutamate, which causes cellular damage and petechial hemorrhages at the injury site. Calcium influx into the neuron is caused by thrombus formation. This alteration in calcium triggers the arachidonic acid cascade, leading to free radical formation, lactic acidosis, and lipid peroxidation. This final series of events hastens ischemia of the white matter and microvasculature destruction, with resultant neuronal damage and permanent neurological deficit.

SCI can be classified by a variety of methods: complete and incomplete cord injury, mechanism of injury, and level of injury. In a complete SCI, the patient loses all function below the neurological injury level (the lowest neurological segment with intact motor and sensory function). In an incomplete SCI, some motor or sensory function below the neurological injury level remains intact. Leading causes of SCI include motor vehicle crashes (MVCs), falls, acts of violence, and sporting injuries.

Where It Occurs

- The majority of acute SCIs occur between the ages of 16 and 18.
- The vast majority, approximately 80%, involve men.

Signal Symptoms

- Permanent and often devastating neurologic deficits and disability; motor and sensory weakness below the level of injury; lack of movement or sensation below the level of injury; lack of urinary and GI sphincter tone.
- Cervical injuries: weak cough; absent, reduced, or limited respiratory effort; poor chest wall expansion; pallor; cyanosis; increased accessory muscle use.
- Autonomic dysfunction: tachycardia, diaphoresis, hypotension.
- Normal sphincter tone and anal winking indicate an incomplete SCI.

BE SAFE! Examine the patient for signs of neurogenic shock, which usually occurs within 30 to 60 minutes after the SCI.

Diagnostic Tests

Test	What It Tells	Patient Problems/ Nursing Care
Spine x-rays	Determines the integrity of bony structures of spine	Knowledge deficit: explain all procedures.
Computed tomography scan	Determines degree and extent of injury	Knowledge deficit: explain all procedures.

Treatment and Nursing Care

Potential Nursing Diagnoses*

Disturbed sensory perception (kinesthetic)
Ineffective airway clearance
Ineffective breathing pattern
Risk for injury
Risk for infection

BE SMART! Patients with a cervical or high thoracic injury are at risk for developing pulmonary insufficiency, problems with airway clearance, and ineffective breathing patterns. Place them in a cervical collar and board before transporting to hospital.

- Early spinal stabilization decreases morbidity and length of hospital stay, but the neurological benefits are controversial.
- Methylprednisolone reduces inflammation and improves motor and sensory function.
- Inotropic agents improve systemic vascular resistance and blood pressure.
- Maintenance of ABCs is the highest nursing priority in patients with SCI.
- Injury level dictates the symptoms. Most patients will need rehabilitation, but the type of rehabilitation depends on the level of injury. Teach patient about sexual function, nutrition, mobility, medications, and treatment options.

Neurological

Stroke

Stroke is the interruption of normal blood flow in one or more of the blood vessels that supply the brain. The tissues become ischemic, leading to hypoxia or anoxia with destruction or necrosis of the neurons, glia, and vasculature. Stroke is the third-leading cause of death in the United States and is an acute neurological injury that occurs because of changes in the blood vessels of the brain. The changes can be intrinsic to the vessel (atherosclerosis, inflammation, arterial dissection, dilation of the vessel, weakening of the vessel, obstruction of the vessel) or extrinsic, such as when an embolism travels from the heart. Although reduced blood flow interferes with brain function, the brain can remain viable with decreased blood flow for long periods of time. However, total cessation of blood flow produces irreversible brain infarction within 3 minutes. Once the blood flow stops, toxins released by damaged neurons, cerebral edema, and alterations in local blood flow contribute to neuron dysfunction and death. Complications of stroke include unstable blood pressure, sensory and motor impairment, infection (encephalitis), pneumonia, contractures, and pulmonary emboli.

Thrombosis, embolism, and hemorrhage are the primary causes of stroke. In cerebral thrombosis, the most common cause of stroke, a blood clot obstructs a cerebral vessel. The most common vessels involved are the carotid arteries of the neck and the arteries in the vertebrobasilar system at the base of the brain near the circle of Willis. Cerebral thrombosis also contributes to transient ischemic attacks (TIAs), which are temporary episodes (10 to 30 minutes) of poor cerebral perfusion caused by partial occlusion of the arterial lumen. A thrombotic stroke that causes a slow evolution of symptoms over several hours is called a *stroke* in evolution. When the condition stabilizes, it is called a *completed stroke*. In an embolic stroke, a clot is carried into the cerebral circulation, usually by the carotid arteries. Blockage of an intracerebral artery results in a localized cerebral infarction. *Hemorrhagic stroke* results from hypertension, rupture of an aneurysm, arteriovenous malformations, or bleeding disorder.

Where It Occurs

■ Risk factors: people with low-density lipoprotein (LDL) and lowered high-density lipoprotein (HDL) levels, people who smoke cigarettes, people who live a sedentary lifestyle.

■ Stroke is considered a complex disease with both genetic and environmental risk factors.

■ Five percent of the population in North America over the age of 65 are affected by stroke.

■ It affects men slightly more often than women and is more common after the age of 50.

■ Blacks/African Americans have a 2.5 times higher rate of stroke than whites.

Signal Symptoms

■ Numbness around the lips and mouth, dizziness, weakness on the affected side, vision deficits (color blindness, lack of depth perception, double vision [diplopia]), poor coordination, difficulty swallowing (dysphagia), slurred speech, amnesia, staggering gait (ataxia).

■ Headache, weakness, paralysis, numbness, sensory changes, altered level of consciousness, bruits over the carotid artery, defective language function (aphasia), speech impairment (dysphasia), eyelid drooping (ptosis).

■ Reading difficulty (dyslexia), visual field deficits, hemiparesis on the affected side (more severe in the face and arm than in the leg).

BE SAFE! Make sure patient has an open airway and can handle secretions; prevent aspiration.

Diagnostic Tests

Test	What It Tells	Patient Problems/ Nursing Care
Computed tomography or magnetic resonance imaging scan	Identification of size and location of site of hemorrhage or infarction	Knowledge deficit: explain all procedures.

Treatment and Nursing Care

Potential Nursing Diagnoses*

Disturbed sensory perception (kinesthetic, visual)
Impaired swallowing
Impaired physical mobility
Anxiety
Ineffective role performance

> **BE SMART!** The treatment needs to be initiated rapidly, within 6 hours of the onset of symptoms.

- Support of vital functions and ongoing surveillance to identify early neurological changes as the patient's condition evolves.
- Therapeutic intervention may save tissue that is at risk for infarction. Recombinant tissue-plasminogen activator (rt-PA) can improve outcome for some patients with acute nonhemorrhagic ischemic stroke if it is given within 3 hours.
- Reduce intracranial pressure (ICP) to limit extension of stroke and prevent complications.
- For patients who cannot maintain airway, breathing, and circulation independently, assist with endotracheal intubation, ventilation, and oxygenation as prescribed. In hemorrhagic stroke, surgery may be required to evacuate a hematoma or to stop bleeding. A ventricular shunt may be placed to drain cerebrospinal fluid.
- Physical therapy is begun as soon as the patient's condition stabilizes. Use passive range-of-motion exercises on the affected side. Strengthening the unaffected side assists the patient in compensating for the losses of the opposite hemisphere.
- The physical therapist teaches the patient to transfer with the use of assistive devices, and the physical or occupational therapist teaches the patient how to perform self-care activity.
- Teach patients all medications, activity restrictions, diet, and self-care activities.

Subarachnoid Hemorrhage

Subarachnoid hemorrhage (SAH) is the direct hemorrhage of arterial blood into the subarachnoid space. Immediately after rupture, intracranial pressure (ICP) rises, resulting in a fall in cerebral perfusion pressure (CPP = mean arterial pressure – ICP). The expanding hematoma acts as a space-occupying lesion, as it compresses or displaces brain tissue. Blood in the subarachnoid space may impede the flow and reabsorption of cerebrospinal fluid (CSF), resulting in hydrocephalus. The bleeding ceases with the formation of a fibrin-platelet plug at the point of the rupture and by tissue compression. As the clot, which forms initially to seal the rupture site, undergoes normal lysis or dissolution, the risk of rebleeding increases.

SAH typically results from cerebral aneurysm rupture (70%), which occurs when the blood vessel wall becomes so thin that it can no longer withstand the surrounding arterial pressure.

Where It Occurs

- Peak incidence of aneurysm rupture is between 40 and 65 years of age.
- Under the age of 40, SAH occurs more commonly in men, but after the age of 50, it is more common in women.
- In the United States, African Americans have a greater risk for SAH than do whites.
- Peak incidence of SAH from arteriovenous malformation is between 30 and 40 years of age.

Signal Symptoms

- Forty-five percent of patients who survive SAH have a sudden, brief loss of consciousness followed by a severe headache.
- Many also report a severe headache associated with exertion but no loss of consciousness.
- Nausea, vomiting, stiff neck, pain in the neck and back, blurred vision, photophobia.

BE SAFE! Make sure the patient has an open airway and adequate breathing.

Diagnostic Tests

Test	What It Tells	Patient Problems/ Nursing Care
Computed tomography scan without contract (urgent)	Identifies areas of bleeding by visualizing any blood collection in subarachnoid space	Knowledge deficit: explain all procedures.

Treatment and Nursing Care

Potential Nursing Diagnoses*

Ineffective tissue perfusion (cerebral)
Pain (acute)
Impaired physical mobility
Disturbed sensory perception (vision)
Anxiety, death

BE SMART! If SAH is managed promptly, some patients have excellent outcomes, but other patients will have irreversible brain damage, and the family may need a great deal of support in making decisions and coping with outcomes.

- Surgery is the treatment of choice for a cerebral aneurysm that has ruptured into the subarachnoid space.
- Nimodipine reduces vasospasm and cerebral ischemia.
- Antihypertensives lower blood pressure but are used only in cases with extreme hypertension.
- Monitoring ICP to detect brain swelling and hydrocephalus and maintaining fluid volume within a normal range are crucial elements of nursing care.
- Rehabilitation is important to help patient regain function and lifestyle. Work with patient and family to achieve the best possible quality of life. If patient has a poor prognosis, discuss options for care and work with the palliative care service to determine best treatment choices.

Subdural Hematoma

Subdural hematoma (SDH) is an accumulating mass of blood, usually clotted, or a swelling that is confined to the space between the dura mater and the subarachnoid membrane. SDHs are space-occupying lesions and thus categorized as focal brain injuries. Sometimes an SDH is called a *mass lesion* because it occupies critical space in the cranial vault. Deaths from SDH usually occur because of the expanding mass lesion that leads to excessive brain swelling and herniation, causing brainstem ischemia and hemorrhage.

SDHs are classified as either acute or chronic on the basis of when symptoms appear. Clinical findings in acute SDHs are evident within 24 to 72 hours after the traumatic event. A subacute SDH produces symptoms within 2 to 10 days; symptoms appear in chronic SDH within weeks or months. The mechanisms of injury associated with the development of SDH are a strong, direct force to the head or an acceleration–deceleration force.

Where It Occurs

- Most head injuries are associated with motor vehicle crashes, which in the 15- to 24-year-old age group are three times more common in males than in females.
- Contact sports are associated with subdural hemotomas.

Signal Symptoms

- Rapidly changing level of consciousness from confusion to coma, ipsilateral pupil dilation, hemiparesis, and abnormal posturing, including flexion and extension.
- Headache, nausea, vomiting, dizziness, convulsions, decreased respiratory rate, or progressive insensitivity to pain (obtundity).

BE SAFE! Patients with SDH may have associated cervical spine injuries or thoracic, abdominal, or extremity trauma.

Diagnostic Tests

Test	What It Tells	Patient Problems/ Nursing Care
Computed tomography scan	Identifies mass lesion	Knowledge deficit: explain all procedures.

Treatment and Nursing Care

Potential Nursing Diagnoses*

Ineffective airway clearance
Risk for aspiration
Risk for acute confusion
Risk for infection
Impaired physical mobility

BE SMART! Begin planning rehabilitation at the time of discharge to ensure the best outcomes.

- Endotracheal intubation and mechanical ventilation are critical to ensure oxygenation and ventilation and to decrease the risk of pulmonary aspiration.
- Surgical management is the evacuation of the clot, control of the hemorrhage, and resection of nonviable brain tissue.
- Diuretics assist in managing intracranial hypertension.
- Sedatives control intermittent increases in intracranial pressure with a resultant decrease in cerebral perfusion pressure.
- The highest priority in managing patients with SDH is to maintain a patent airway, appropriate ventilation and oxygenation, and adequate circulation.
- Upon discharge, the patient will likely need rehabilitation, patient and family teaching, and careful discharge planning.

Transient Ischemic Attack

Transient ischemic attack (TIA) is a sudden onset of temporary neurologic dysfunction caused by microemboli or decreased perfusion in either the carotid or vertebrobasilar circulations. The TIA resolves without residual deficit in less than 24 hours (usually within 1 to 2 hours from onset) or by platelet aggregates that form on atheromatous plaques and embolize to occlude a distal arteriole temporarily. A TIA is considered prognostic for stroke; 15% of strokes are preceded by TIAs.

In adults, causes include atherosclerosis of carotid and vertebral arteries, tumors, emboli from valvular disease, illicit drugs such as cocaine, arterial dissection, cerebral events such as subdural hematomas. People with recent cardiac or carotid surgery, seizures, central nervous system and sinus infections, and thromboembolism are predisposed to TIAs.

Where It Occurs

- Typically occurs in patients older than 45, with highest incidence after the age of 70.
- Men are three times more likely than women to suffer a TIA.

Signal Symptoms

- Diplopia, vertigo, ataxia, facial paresis, Horner's syndrome, dysphagia, dysarthria, and blurred vision.
- Ocular changes, incomplete closure of eyelids, visual defects, asymmetrical mouth, poor shoulder shrugging.
- Motor and sensory deficits.

BE SAFE! Rapid transportation to a hospital for evaluation of the symptoms is critical.

Diagnostic Tests

Test	What It Tells	Patient Problems/ Nursing Care
Prothrombin time/partial thromboplastin time	Suggests hypercoagulopathies	Knowledge deficit: explain procedures. Patient will need venipuncture.
Duplex carotid scan	Shows carotid stenosis	Knowledge deficit: explain procedures.

Treatment and Nursing Care

Potential Nursing Diagnoses*

Ineffective tissue perfusion (cerebral)
Activity intolerance
Impaired memory
Impaired physical mobility

BE SMART! Make sure the patient understands the side effects of anticoagulant therapy.

- Anticoagulant and antiplatelet medications can abolish TIAS.
- If surgery is pursued, carotid endarterectomy may be performed.
- Manage hypertension.
- Nursing care involves encouraging rest, teaching about medications and other prevention strategies, and activity recommendations.

Traumatic Brain Injury

Traumatic brain injury (TBI) is an insult to the brain from an external force that may lead to permanent or temporary neurological dysfunction. Severity of brain injury can be determined using various measures, such as eye opening, motor response, and verbal response. Injuries are classified as either primary or secondary depending on whether they occur at the time of trauma or immediately after. They are also classified as blunt (acceleration or deceleration force that damages the contents of the cranium) or penetrating (a projectile breaches the cranium but does not exit it) depending on the nature of the injury. Motor vehicle crashes (MVCs) are the most common cause of TBIs.

Where It Occurs

- Most head injuries are associated with MVCs, which in the 15- to 24-year-old age group are three times more common in males than in females.
- Contact sports are associated with blunt TBI.
- Penetrating TBI is associated with assaults with weapons. Gunshot wound is most common.

Signal Symptoms

- May have no change in consciousness to rapidly changing level of consciousness; confusion to coma; ipsilateral pupil dilation; hemiparesis; and abnormal posturing, including flexion and extension.
- Headache, nausea, vomiting, dizziness, convulsions, decreased respiratory rate, or progressive insensitivity to pain (obtundity).
- Open head wound of varying sizes with bleeding or oozing.

BE SAFE! Patients with TBI may have associated cervical spine injuries or thoracic, abdominal, or extremity trauma.

Diagnostic Tests

Test	What It Tells	Patient Problems/ Nursing Care
Computed tomography scan	Identifies mass lesion	Knowledge deficit: explain all procedures.

Treatment and Nursing Care

Potential Nursing Diagnoses*

Ineffective airway clearance
Risk for aspiration

Pain (acute)
Risk for acute confusion
Risk for infection
Impaired physical mobility

BE SMART! Begin planning rehabilitation at the time of discharge to ensure the best outcomes.

- Endotracheal intubation and mechanical ventilation are critical to ensure oxygenation and ventilation and to decrease the risk of pulmonary aspiration. The highest priority in managing patients with TBI is to maintain a patent airway, appropriate ventilation and oxygenation, and adequate circulation.
- Surgical management may be needed to manage a penetrating missile, evacuate a clot, control hemorrhage, or resect nonviable brain tissue.
- Diuretics assist in managing intracranial hypertension.
- Sedatives control intermittent increases in intracranial pressure with a resultant decrease in cerebral perfusion pressure. Analgesics are needed to manage pain.
- Upon discharge, the patient will likely need rehabilitation, patient and family teaching, and careful discharge planning.

Adrenal Insufficiency

Adrenal insufficiency can be primary or secondary. Addison's disease, primary adrenal insufficiency, occurs rarely with lack of hormone production by the adrenal gland. Secondary insufficiency occurs from disorders of the pituitary gland. The adrenal glands consist of the medulla and the cortex. The medulla is responsible for the secretion of the catecholamines epinephrine and norepinephrine; the cortex is responsible for the secretion of glucocorticoids, mineralocorticoids, and androgen. The principal glucocorticoid, cortisol, helps regulate blood pressure, metabolism, anti-inflammatory response, and emotional behavior. The principal mineralocorticoid, aldosterone, is important for regulating sodium levels.

Adrenal insufficiency is characterized by the decreased production of cortisol, aldosterone, and androgen. Cortisol deficiency causes altered metabolism, decreased stress tolerance, and emotional lability. Aldosterone deficiency causes urinary loss of sodium, chloride, and water, resulting in dehydration and electrolyte imbalances. Androgen deficiency leads to the loss of secondary sex characteristics.

Where It Occurs

- Addison's disease, particularly idiopathic autoimmune Addison's disease, affects females more than males and occurs in adults in midlife from ages 30 to 60 years.
- Ethnicity and race do not appear to change the risk for Addison's disease.

Signal Symptoms

- Poor tolerance for stress, weakness, fatigue, and activity.
- Anorexia, nausea, vomiting, or diarrhea.

BE SAFE! Observe for fluid deficit, evidenced by signs of dehydration (tachycardia, weak peripheral pulses, decreased skin turgor, dry mouth).

Diagnostic Tests

Test	What It Tells	Patient Problems/ Nursing Care
Serum cortisol level	Determines the ability of the adrenal gland to produce glucocorticoids	Knowledge deficit: explain procedures. Patient will need venipuncture.
Serum electrolytes and chemistries	Values reflect sodium loss from a deficit in mineralocorticoids with loss of fluids and poor glucose control because of decreased gluconeogenesis	Knowledge deficit: explain procedures. Patient will need venipuncture.

Treatment and Nursing Care

Potential Nursing Diagnoses*

Fluid volume deficit, hypertonic
Altered nutrition, less than body requirements
Ineffective tissue perfusion (cerebral, peripheral)
Risk for unstable blood glucose
Knowledge deficit (medications)

BE SMART! Check for postural hypotension (drop in systolic blood pressure going from a lying to sitting or standing position).

- Collaborative treatment of adrenal insufficiency focuses on restoring fluid, electrolyte, and hormone balances.
- Glucocorticoids such as hydrocortisone, dexamethasone, and prednisone are used as replacement therapy in a deficiency state.
- Fludrocortisone is used as replacement therapy in a deficiency state.
- Nursing care should emphasize education and stress management.

Pancreatic cancer includes carcinomas of the head of the pancreas, the ampulla of Vater, the common bile duct, and the duodenum. Tumors can develop in both the exocrine and the endocrine tissue of the pancreas, although 95% arise from the exocrine parenchyma (functional tissue) and are called *adenocarcinomas*. The remaining 5% of pancreatic tumors develop from endocrine cells of the pancreas; they are named according to the hormone they produce (i.e., insulinomas, glucagonomas).

Adenocarcinoma of the ductal origin is the most common exocrine cell type (75–92%), and it occurs most frequently in the head of the pancreas. Pancreatic adenocarcinoma grows rapidly, spreading to the stomach, duodenum, gallbladder, liver, and intestine by direct extension and invasion of lymphatic and vascular systems. Further metastatic spread to the lung, peritoneum, and spleen can occur. Metastatic tumors from cancers in the lung, breast, thyroid, or kidney or skin melanoma have been found in the pancreas. The overall 5–year survival rate is approximately 5%.

Where It Occurs

- Pancreatic carcinoma can occur in persons of all ages but is rare before the age of 45 and has peak incidence between the ages of 60 and 70.
- Pancreatic cancer occurs 50% more frequently among African Americans than among European Americans, with the highest incidence in the United States developing among Korean Americans living in Los Angeles.

Signal Symptoms

- Early stages: vague symptoms that are frequently disregarded or attributed to a minor ailment.
- Unplanned weight loss and epigastric pain that may radiate to the back are common.

- Jaundice is the presenting symptom in 80% to 90% of patients with cancer of the pancreatic head.
- Late: abdominal pain.

BE SAFE! Healthy lifestyle with avoidance of smoking and overweight/obesity may be protective.

Diagnostic Tests

Test	What It Tells	Patient Problems/ Nursing Care
Computed tomography (CT) scan	Identifies size and location of tumors	Knowledge deficit: explain all procedures.
Magnetic resonance imaging	Identifies size and location of tumors and determines if vessels are compressed by tumor	Knowledge deficit: explain all procedures.

Treatment and Nursing Care

Potential Nursing Diagnoses*

Pain (chronic and acute)
Imbalanced nutrition, less than body requirements
Anxiety, death
Disturbed body image

BE SMART! Because long-term prognosis is poor, the patient and family might consider planning for palliative care.

- Surgery, radiotherapy, and chemotherapy are the major treatment modalities for pancreatic cancer.
- Pancreatic enzyme supplements aid in digestion of proteins, carbohydrates, and fats.
- Nursing care involves providing emotional support after diagnosis, and postoperative care if surgery is performed.

Cancer, Thyroid

Cancer of the thyroid gland is the most common endocrine cancer. Most thyroid nodules or tumors develop from thyroid follicular cells; 95% of these nodules and tumors are benign. The remaining 5% of thyroid nodules or tumors are cancerous, and there are several forms of thyroid cancer. Papillary carcinoma is the most common form of primary thyroid cancer. It is also the slowest-growing thyroid cancer and is usually multifocal and bilateral in distribution. Papillary carcinoma metastasizes slowly into the cervical lymph nodes and the nodes of the mediastinum and lungs. Follicular cancer is the next most common form. It is more likely to recur than other forms; it generally metastasizes to the regional lymph nodes and is spread by the blood to distant areas such as the bones, liver, and lungs.

Anaplastic carcinoma of the thyroid is a less common form of thyroid cancer and is resistant to both surgical resection and radiation.

Where It Occurs

- Although benign thyroid nodules and thyroid cancers can occur in people of all ages, those between 30 and 50 years old are most likely to develop papillary and follicular thyroid cancer.
- Women are three times as likely as men to have thyroid cancer.
- There is a genetic link to thyroid cancer as well as a link to radiation accidents.

Signal Symptoms

- Most common: asymptomatic neck mass.
- Neck discomfort, hoarseness, dysphagia, feeling as if "breathing through a straw," persistent cough, stridor, vocal cord paralysis, hemoptysis, and rapid nodule growth.

BE SAFE! Airway blockage is the most serious complication from tumor growth and complications of surgery.

Diagnostic Tests

Test	What It Tells	Patient Problems/ Nursing Care
Fine-needle aspiration (FNA) biopsy	Microscopic viewing reveals cancer cells	Knowledge deficit: explain procedures. Check for bleeding and infection at biopsy site.
Thyroid scan	Abnormal areas of the thyroid may contain less radioactivity (cold nodules with decreased uptake)	Knowledge deficit: explain procedures.

Treatment and Nursing Care

Potential Nursing Diagnoses*

Ineffective airway clearance
Ineffective breathing pattern
Knowledge deficit (medications, surgery, postoperative care, surveillance)
Anxiety

> **BE SMART!** Changes in thyroid function may also lead to gastrointestinal changes such as diarrhea and anorexia.

- Most physicians prescribe surgical treatment of thyroid cancer; the definitive treatment depends on the size of the nodule.
- Surgical interventions range from a thyroid lobectomy for cancers smaller than 1 cm that show no signs of metastasis to a total thyroidectomy and, possibly, a modified neck dissection if lymph nodes need to be removed.

- Levothyroxine (Synthroid) suppresses TSH levels and establishes a euthyroid state postoperatively.
- The most important nursing interventions focus on teaching and prevention of complications.

Cushing's Syndrome

Cushing's syndrome is the clinical effects of increased exposure to glucocorticoid hormone. It can be characterized by an excess production of glucocorticoids (primarily cortisol) by the cortex of the adrenal gland, but it is most commonly due to therapy with glucocorticoid medications.

Overproduction of glucocorticoids leads to a host of multisystem disorders in metabolism, water balance, wound healing, and response to infection. Complications affect almost every system of the body. Increased calcium resorption from bones may lead to osteoporosis and bone fractures. A blunted immune response causes a high risk for infection as well as poor wound healing. Cushing's syndrome may also mask life-threatening infections. Gastrointestinal (GI) irritation may lead to peptic ulcers, and both insulin resistance and glucose intolerance can cause hyperglycemia.

Where It Occurs

- In adults, secondary Cushing's syndrome that results from pituitary disease is most common in females age 30 to 50 years.
- Secondary disease is more common than primary disease in children older than 6 or 7.
- Secondary Cushing's syndrome that results from increased adrenocorticotrophic hormone (ACTH) secretion, particularly from lung tumors, is more common in males.

Signal Symptoms

- Classic signs are a moon-shaped face, fat pads at the upper back (supraclavicular fat pads and buffalo hump), truncal obesity, thin extremities, and purple lines or striae of the skin.

■ Changes in memory, attention span, or behavior; muscle weakness; weight gain; increased body hair.

■ Sleep disturbances, weakness, fatigue, back pain, general discomfort, difficulty completing activities of daily living, and changes in the urinary output.

BE SAFE! Although Cushing's syndrome is usually due to glucocorticoid administration, pituitary and adrenal tumors and other conditions can also cause it and should be ruled out, particularly in people 25 to 40 years of age.

Diagnostic Tests

Test	What It Tells	Patient Problems/ Nursing Care
Overnight dexamethasone suppression test	Elevated levels due to a failure to suppress normal cortisol response is diagnostic of Cushing's syndrome	Knowledge deficit: explain all procedures. Patient will need venipuncture.
Low-dose dexamathasone suppression test	Elevated levels due to a failure to suppress normal cortisol response is diagnostic of Cushing's syndrome	Knowledge deficit: explain all procedures. Patient will need venipuncture.

Treatment and Nursing Care

Potential Nursing Diagnoses*

Fluid volume excess
Impaired tissue integrity
Fatigue
Imbalanced nutrition, potential for more than body requirements
Risk for infection
Risk for injury

BE SMART! Corticosteroids should be withdrawn gradually to prevent adrenal crisis.

- The main focus is to find the primary cause of the cortisol excess and remove it if possible. If a tumor is present, resection of the tumor if possible. Some patients will receive radiation.
- Mitotane inhibits activity of adrenal cortex but is used with caution.
- Cyproheptadine inhibits the release of ACTH from pituitary gland but is used only as a last resort.
- Assess the patient for an unsteady gait; falls and fractures are common due to accompanying osteoporosis.
- Nursing care focuses on limiting the risk of infection, and postoperative care if surgery is performed.

Diabetes Mellitus, Type 1

Diabetes mellitus (DM) is a chronic disorder of carbohydrate, protein, and fat metabolism in which there is a discrepancy between the amount of insulin required by the body and the amount of insulin available. In type 1, or *insulin-dependent diabetes mellitus*, patients are dependent on insulin for prevention of hyperglycemia or ketosis. The beta cells of the pancreas produce insulin and a protein called C-peptide, which are stored in the secretory granules of the beta cells and are released into the bloodstream as blood glucose levels increase. Insulin transports glucose and amino acids across the membranes of many body cells, particularly muscle and fat cells. It also increases the liver storage of glycogen, the chief carbohydrate storage material, and aids in the metabolism of triglycerides, nucleic acids, and proteins. In type 1 DM, the pancreas cannot release insulin, leading to absent or low levels of circulating insulin, elevation of plasma glucagon, and lack of response by pancreatic beta cells to insulin-secretory stimuli.

A common theory explaining the cause of type 1 DM is that infectious or environmental agents damage the pancreas or lead to autoimmunity. Possible triggers include cow's milk, viruses such as rubella, or toxic chemicals. Type 1 DM is also associated with other autoimmune diseases such as Graves' disease, Hashimoto thyroiditis, and Addison's disease.

Where It Occurs

- Type 1 DM most commonly develops in childhood before age 20 but can occur at any age. In adults, it is most typically diagnosed in the third or fourth decade of life.
- Whites are more typically affected with type 1 DM than are other groups. Unlike type 2 DM, type 1 DM does not generally occur in people who are obese.
- Type 1 DM is often diagnosed when a lean patient experiences diabetic ketoacidosis.

Signal Symptoms

- Polyuria, polydipsia, and polyphagia are the classic signs of type 1 DM. Other signs are fatigue (often considered the most common sign), lassitude, nausea, abdominal discomfort, weight loss, and blurred vision.
- Dehydration, muscle cramping.

BE SAFE! Type 1 DM may have a sudden onset and may occur along with an infectious process that presents an unusual stressor to the body. Symptoms need rapid attention to prevent diabetic ketoacidosis.

Diagnostic Tests

Test	What It Tells	Patient Problems/ Nursing Care
Fasting plasma glucose (FPG)	Elevated levels of glucose because insufficient insulin is available to transport insulin into body cells	Knowledge deficit: explain procedures. Patient will need venipuncture.
Glycosylated hemoglobin (Hb A_{1c})	Elevated over 6.5%; reflects the average glucose over the last 4–12 weeks as measured by Hb A_{1c}; shows exposure of hemoglobin to glucose in the blood	Knowledge deficit: explain procedures. Patient will need venipuncture.

Treatment and Nursing Care

Potential Nursing Diagnoses*

Imbalanced nutrition, less than body requirements
Fluid volume deficit
Risk for unstable blood glucose
Knowledge deficit (medications, nutrition, physical activity, glucose
  regulation, health-care follow-up)
Risk for infection

BE SMART! Help the patient institute treatment promptly. Some
patients have significant weight loss and wasting, depending on
the time between the onset of the disease and treatment.

- DM has no known cure, and management of the disease focuses
  control of the serum glucose level to prevent or delay the
  development of complications.
- Individuals with type 1 DM require subcutaneous insulin
  administration to replace deficient or absent levels.
- Antidiabetics may also be used as an alternative to insulin.
- Tight glucose control with a premeal glucose level of 80 to
  130 mg/dL or Hb A_{1c} less than 7% is considered by some experts as
  ideal. Advances in technology for glucose monitoring and insulin
  delivery systems (continuous subcutaneous insulin administration)
  enable tight glucose control for many patients.
- Significant complications generally occur over the diabetic's life
  and need to be managed. These include peripheral neuropathy,
  microvascular complications (retinopathy and nephropathy),
  macrovascular complications such as hypertension, foot ulcers,
  and both hyperglycemia and hypoglycemia.
- Education is the most important part of diabetes management.
  Content is critical and includes explanations of diabetes itself and
  the long-term course of the disease; self-management including diet,
  insulin administration, and blood glucose monitoring; and long-term
  complications. Teaching about the signs, symptoms, and management
  of hypoglycemia are important.

Diabetes Mellitus, Type 2

Diabetes mellitus (DM) is a chronic disorder of carbohydrate, protein, and fat metabolism in which there is a discrepancy between the amount of insulin required by the body and the amount of insulin available. In type 2 DM, or *non-insulin-dependent diabetes mellitus*, patients are usually not initially dependent on insulin but have either insulin resistance or impaired insulin secretion. As the disease evolves, however, they may become dependent on insulin. In type 2 DM, relative insulin deficiency (compared to the absolute insulin deficiency in type 1 DM) is accompanied by resistance to the actions of insulin in muscle, fat, and liver cells.

Where It Occurs

- Type 2 DM usually occurs after the age of 30, particularly in individuals who are overweight, obese, or have hereditary factors.
- Patients who are diagnosed with type 2 diabetes typically have had diabetes for at least 4 years.
- Type 2 DM is more common in Native Americans, Hispanics, and African Americans than in whites, but the incidence is equal in females and males in all populations.
- DM incidence increases with age.

Signal Symptoms

- Polyuria, polydipsia, and polyphagia are the classic signs of DM.
- Fatigue, lassitude, nausea, vomiting, abdominal discomfort.
- Itching, blurred vision, and frequent infections are common complaints in individuals with type 2 DM. A common symptom of DM is fatigue, but patients with type 2 DM may not report this symptom.

BE SAFE! **The goal of patients with type 2 DM is to slow the progression of the disease and limit the chance of complications.**

Diagnostic Tests

Test	What It Tells	Patient Problems/ Nursing Care
Fasting plasma glucose (FPG)	Elevated levels because insufficient insulin is available to transport insulin into body cells	Knowledge deficit: explain procedures. Patient will need venipuncture.
Glycosylated hemoglobin (Hb A_{1c})	Elevated over 6.5%; reflects the average glucose over the last 4–12 weeks as measured by Hb A_{1c}; shows exposure of hemoglobin to glucose in the blood	Knowledge deficit: explain procedures. Patient will need venipuncture.

Treatment and Nursing Care

Potential Nursing Diagnoses*

Imbalanced nutrition, more than body requirements
Risk for unstable blood glucose
Knowledge deficit (medications, nutrition, physical activity, glucose regulation, health-care follow-up)
Risk for infection

BE SMART! The patient with type 2 DM may have thin limbs with fatty deposits around the face, neck, and abdomen.

- DM has no known cure, and management of the disease focuses on control of the serum glucose level to prevent or delay the development of complications.
- Patients with type 2 DM may be able to control the disease by diet management and weight reduction, if necessary.
- Exenatide (Byetta) is used to improve glycemic control for type 2 diabetics.
- Significant complications generally occur over the diabetic's life and need to be managed. These include peripheral neuropathy,

microvascular complications (retinopathy and nephropathy), macrovascular complications such as hypertension, foot ulcers, and both hyperglycemia and hypoglycemia.
- Nursing care focuses on explaining the disease process and explaining disease management to the patient.

Diabetic Ketoacidosis

Diabetic ketoacidosis (DKA) is an acute and serious complication of diabetes that more commonly occurs in patients with type 1 diabetes mellitus (DM) but also occurs with type 2 DM. It is characterized by an absolute or relative deficiency in insulin that is exacerbated by consequent hyperglycemia, dehydration, acidosis, ketosis, and other metabolic dysfunctions. The most common causes are underlying infection, disruption of insulin treatment, and new onset of diabetes. DKA has a relatively strict biochemical profile: ketones greater than 5 mEq/L, blood glucose level greater than 250 mg/dL, and an arterial blood pH less than 7.3.

DKA is typically caused by an intercurrent condition such as myocardial infarction, infection, sepsis, stroke, insulin treatment disruption, and recent development of diabetes.

Where It Occurs

- DKA occurs more often in whites because of their higher propensity for type 1 DM.
- Women suffer from DKA at a slightly higher rate than men.

Signal Symptoms

- Polydipsia and polyuria are the most frequent early symptoms.
- Mental status changes occur in direct proportion to the levels of dehydration and hyperglycemia; the higher the glucose, the less alert the patient.
- Weakness, fatigue, malaise, nausea, vomiting, abdominal pain, anorexia.
- Late: dry mucous membranes, ketone "fruity" breath, decreased reflexes, hypotension, tachycardia.

BE SAFE! If DKA has progressed, observe that the patient has a
patent airway with good gas exchange.

Diagnostic Tests

Test	What It Tells	Patient Problems/ Nursing Care
Blood test for glucose	Increased levels indicate hyperglycemia	Knowledge deficit: explain procedures. Patient will need venipuncture.
Glycosylated hemoglobin (Hb A_{1c})	Elevated over 6.5%; reflects the average glucose over the last 4–12 weeks as measured by Hb A_{1c}; shows exposure of hemoglobin to glucose in the blood	Knowledge deficit: explain procedures. Patient will need venipuncture.
Arterial pH	Decreased levels reflect accumulation of hydrogen ions and acidosis	Knowledge deficit: explain procedures. Patient will need arterial puncture.

Treatment and Nursing Care

Potential Nursing Diagnoses*

Risk for unstable blood glucose
Risk for ineffective airway clearance
Imbalanced nutrition
Risk for fluid volume deficit

BE SMART! Evaluate the patient's knowledge and determine if
patient needs more education about prevention.

- Generally, IV insulin supplementation is necessary. Observe for rapid
drops in glucose. A slow, progressively decreasing blood glucose
prevents rebound hypoglycemia and hypokalemia.

- Restoring fluid and electrolyte balance is a crucial element to treating DKA.
- Manage concurrent conditions such as myocardial infarction and infection.
- Evaluate the patient's teaching needs (medications, nutrition, physical activity, hydration).

Hyperglycemia

Hyperglycemia exists when the fasting blood glucose level is greater than 110 mg/dL or a 2-hour postprandial level is above 140 mg/dL. Prediabetes occurs when blood glucose levels are higher than normal but not high enough for a diagnosis of diabetes. This condition is sometimes called impaired fasting glucose or impaired glucose tolerance.

Insulin is produced by the beta cells of the pancreas, which are stimulated to release it when the blood glucose level rises. Insulin transports glucose, amino acids, potassium, and phosphate across the cell membrane. Insufficient production or ineffective use of insulin causes an elevated blood glucose level (hyperglycemia), which promotes water movement into the bloodstream from the interstitial space and intracellular fluid compartments. As blood glucose levels increase, the renal threshold for glucose reabsorption is exceeded, and glycosuria (loss of glucose in the urine) occurs. Glucose in the urine acts as an osmotic diuretic, and the patient has an increased urinary output in response that can lead to a serious fluid volume deficit. As glucose levels climb, the blood becomes more viscous and the patient is also at risk for thromboembolic phenomena. The two primary causes of hyperglycemia are diabetes mellitus and hyperosmolar nonketotic syndrome (HNKS).

Where It Occurs

- Although there are no racial or ethnic considerations for hyperglycemia, there are different patterns of types 1 and 2 DM across populations.
- Type 1 DM most commonly develops in childhood before age 20 but can occur at any age.
- Type 2 DM usually occurs after the age of 30, particularly in individuals who are overweight, obese, or have hereditary factors.

Signal Symptoms

- Polyuria and polydipsia.
- Unless the blood glucose level has increased enough to cause fluid volume deficit and dehydration, symptoms may not be present.

BE SAFE! If hyperglycemia goes without correction, dehydration, mental status changes, and diabetic ketoacidosis might occur.

Diagnostic Tests

Test	What It Tells	Patient Problems/ Nursing Care
Serum glucose level (fasting)	Elevation of glucose resulting from insulin deficit, insulin resistance, or pancreatic disease	Knowledge deficit: explain procedures. Patient will need venipuncture.
Serum osmolarity	Reflects increased concentration of particles in extracellular fluid	Knowledge deficit: explain procedures. Patient will need venipuncture.

Treatment and Nursing Care

Potential Nursing Diagnoses*

Risk for unstable blood glucose
Fluid volume deficit
Nutrition, imbalanced, more than body requirements
Risk for infection

BE SMART! Embolic events are possible from dehydration, sluggish circulation, and increased coagulation. Assess for signs of pulmonary embolus.

- If the serum glucose level is above 250 mg/dL and the fluid balance is adequate, insulin is usually prescribed either as a subcutaneous injection or as an IV push injection or an intravenous drip.

- If a patient has an elevated serum glucose along with a fluid volume deficit, the fluid volume deficit is corrected before the glucose excess.
- Observe the patient for hypokalemia as you lower the blood glucose.
- The first nursing priority is to maintain adequate fluid balance. Assess mental status regularly and watch for rebound hypoglycemia (lightheadedness, tachycardia, diaphoresis, syncope, nausea).
- Assess the patient's level of knowledge and provide medication and nutritional teaching as needed.

Hyperglycemic Hyperosmolar Nonketotic Coma (HHNC)

Hyperosmolar hyperglycemic state (HHS) is a metabolic dysfunction characterized by hyperglycemia, hyperosmolarity, and dehydration. It is an acute metabolic complication of diabetes mellitus (DM) with the following criteria: serum osmolality of 320 mOsm/kg, plasma glucose level greater than 600 mg/dL (>33.3 mmol/L), profound dehydration, no ketoacidosis, pH of 7.3, HCO_3- greater than 15 mEq/L, and the absence of severe ketosis. It is often the initial presentation of patients with type 2 DM. It may be associated with stressful physiological conditions such as infection, sepsis, myocardial infarction, or stroke.

Where It Occurs

- HHS typically is found in older patients with type 2 DM.
- Type 2 DM usually occurs after the age of 30, particularly in individuals who are overweight, obese, or have hereditary factors.

Signal Symptoms

- Possible symptoms include polydipsia, polyuria, weight loss, and weakness.
- Neurological issues may also be found, such as delirium or sensory deficits.
- Unless the blood glucose level has increased enough to cause fluid volume deficit and dehydration, symptoms may not be present.

BE SAFE! Observe for decreased mental status; if mental status decreases, make sure the patient has a patent airway and adequate breathing.

Diagnostic Tests

Test	What It Tells	Patient Problems/ Nursing Care
Blood glucose level	Elevated levels indicate hyperglycemia	Knowledge deficit: explain procedures. Patient will need venipuncture.

Treatment and Nursing Care

Potential Nursing Diagnoses*

Risk for unstable blood glucose
Fluid volume deficit
Nutrition, imbalanced, more than body requirements
Risk for infection

BE SMART! Embolic events are possible from dehydration, sluggish circulation, and increased coagulation. Assess for signs of pulmonary embolus.

- Fluid and electrolyte replacement are crucial elements to treating HHS.
- Hydrate and bring the blood glucose down slowly to prevent fluid shifts and central nervous system changes. Insulin is usually prescribed either as a subcutaneous injection or as an IV push injection or an intravenous drip. Replace potassium as glucose is decreased.
- Generally an indwelling urinary catheter is necessary to monitor fluid volume status.
- Assess the patient for underlying disease processes.
- Provide diabetes education.

Myxedema

Myxedema coma is a life-threatening state characterized by cardio-vascular collapse, severe electrolyte imbalances, respiratory depression, and cerebral hypoxia. It is the most severe but rare form of hypothyroidism and occurs when it is either undertreated or not diagnosed.

Hypothyroidism is usually an autoimmune response but may also be due to iodine deficiency. When no thyroid hormone is present, deficits occur in cell metabolism and organ function, leading to inadequate nutrition, maturation of tissues, and energy production. Overdosing on medications such as opiates, anesthetic agents, and sedatives is associated with myxedema crisis.

Where It Occurs

- Women over age 60 are more likely than other populations to develop myxedema.
- Patients who progress rapidly from hypothyroidism to myxedema have conditions such as stroke, multiple trauma, gastrointestinal hemorrhage, heart failure, or bacterial infection.
- Often occurs during winter months.

Signal Symptoms

- Fatigue, activity intolerance, weight gain, intolerance to cold, dry skin, constipation, mental sluggishness, thinning hair.
- Lethargy, delirium, coma.

BE SAFE! If patient is unresponsive, obtain a health history from the family and ask specifically about changes in mental status, weight gain, and cold intolerance.

Diagnostic Tests

Test	What It Tells	Patient Problems/ Nursing Care
Free thyroxine (T4) and thyroid-stimulating hormone (TSH)	Decreased free T4 levels and elevated or decreased TSH levels indicate thyroid disorder	Knowledge deficit: explain procedures. Patient will need venipuncture.
Serum electrolytes and serum osmolality	Hyponatremia with low serum osmolality is consistent with a diagnosis of myxedema	Knowledge deficit: explain procedures. Patient will need venipuncture.

Treatment and Nursing Care

Potential Nursing Diagnoses*

Inadequate airway clearance
Risk for infection
Risk for injury
Risk for aspiration
Hypothermia

BE SMART! Teach the patient or family that thyroid medications are necessary for supplementation for life.

- Mechanical ventilation may be necessary.
- Thyroid hormone replacement may be implemented intravenously.
- Following obtaining a cortisol level, corticosteroids may be administered. Manage infection and correct fluid and electrolyte imbalances such as hyponatremia and hypovolemia.
- Supportive care such as help with hygiene, maintaining a patent airway, and nutritional supplementation are important.

Obesity Surgery

Bariatric surgery is the only known procedure to result in significant and sustained weight loss in morbidly obese patients (people with a body mass index [BMI] of 40 kg/m^2 or more). Bariatric surgery is based on three basic ideas: gastric restriction, gastric restriction with mild malabsorption, and mild gastric restriction in combination with malabsorption. Most procedures are done through laparoscopic procedures and include horizontal gastroplasty, gastric banding, Roux-en-Y gastric bypass, biliopancreatic bypass, and jejunoileal bypass procedures.

Bariatric surgery improves or resolves many weight-related conditions such as type 2 diabetes mellitus, hypertension, and heart failure; asthma, esophagitis, sleep disorder; osteoarthritis; and urinary incontinence.

Where It Occurs

- BMI indicating obesity of 30 kg/m^2 or more.
- Waist circumference more than 35 inches in women or 40 inches in men.
- Up to 70% of the U.S. population is overweight, and half of this group are obese. Up to 25% of children in the United States are obese.
- More women than men are obese in the United States.
- Ethnic groups native to North America have a particularly high prevalence of obesity. In addition, Polynesians, Micronesians, Anurans, Maoris of the West and East Indies, African Americans in North America, and the Hispanic populations (both Mexican and Puerto Rican in origin) in North America also have particularly high predispositions to developing obesity.

Signal Symptoms

- Morbid obesity.
- Shortness of breath on exertion, hypertension, peripheral edema, glycosuria, joint pain, disordered sleep, epigastric burning.

BE SAFE! A thorough evaluation is needed by an anesthesiologist before surgery because of the high-risk population.

Diagnostic Tests

Test	What It Tells	Patient Problems/ Nursing Care
BMI	Calculated by dividing weight in kilograms by height in meters, squared. Normal BMI = 18.5–24.9 kg/m^2; overweight is BMI = 25–29.9 kg/m^2; obese is BMI 30 kg/m^2 or more	Knowledge deficit: explain procedures.

Treatment and Nursing Care

Potential Nursing Diagnoses*

Nutrition, imbalance, more than body requirements
Activity intolerance
Risk for infection
Anxiety
Ineffective coping

BE SMART! Observe carefully for surgical complications such as bleeding, infection, and thromboembolism.

- Preoperative and postoperative nutritional counseling is critical. Some patients may be placed on a restrictive diet before surgery to reduce the size of the liver and to determine the success of postoperative nutritional changes.
- Surgical body contouring is often needed to manage flabby skin and abdominal overhang.
- Observe for complications such as anastomotic leaks, emboli and thrombi, infection, gastrointestinal bleed, and pneumonia.
- Teach patients how to manage dietary restrictions, portion size, foods to avoid. Provide referral to consultations for depression or difficulty with managing body image issues and lifestyle changes.

Pancreatitis

Pancreatitis, acute or chronic, is an inflammation and potential necrosis of the pancreas. Tissue damage from pancreatitis occurs because of activation of proteolytic and lipolytic pancreatic enzymes that are normally activated in the duodenum. Proteolytic enzymes, such as trypsin, elastase, and phospholipase, break down protein; lipolytic enzymes break down fats. The enzymes cause autodigestion (destruction of the acinar cells and islet cell tissue), with leakage of the enzymes and fluid into surrounding tissues. The pancreas can return to normal after an attack of acute pancreatitis with successful treatment, or it may progress to a state of chronic inflammation and disease.

In chronic pancreatitis, permanent destruction occurs. Precipitation of proteins causes pancreatic duct obstruction. Edema and distention cause damage and loss of the acinar cells, which normally produce digestive enzymes. The normal cells are replaced with fibrosis and necrosis. As the autodigestion process of the pancreas progresses, the cells form walls around the fluid that contains enzymes and the necrotic debris. These pseudocysts can rupture into the peritoneum and surrounding tissues, resulting in complications of infection, abscesses, and fistulae.

Where It Occurs

■ The risk for middle-aged African Americans is 10 times higher than that of whites and Native Americans, and the racial/ethnic differences are more pronounced in men than in women.
■ More men than women have pancreatitis.
■ Pancreatitis is associated with alcohol misuse and dependence, injury, drugs, AIDS, and vasculitis.

Signal Symptoms

■ Upper abdominal pain described as knifelike, twisting, and deep in the midepigastrium or umbilical region is common.
■ Nausea, vomiting, anorexia, diarrhea.
■ Restlessness, apprehension, and agitated behavior.

BE SAFE! People with pancreatitis need careful monitoring. They can progress rapidly from symptoms of abdominal pain to shock and sepsis.

Diagnostic Tests

Test	What It Tells	Patient Problems/ Nursing Care
Serum amylase	Enzyme produced by pancreas that aids digestion of complex carbohydrates and increases 12–24 hours after acute inflammation	Knowledge deficit: explain procedures. Patient will need venipuncture.
Serum calcium	Necrosis of fat from release of pancreatic enzymes leads to binding of free calcium	Knowledge deficit: explain procedures. Patient will need venipuncture.

Treatment and Nursing Care

Potential Nursing Diagnoses*

Pain (acute or chronic)
Nausea
Diarrhea
Imbalanced nutrition, less than body requirements
Fluid volume deficit
Risk for infection

BE SMART! Electrolyte imbalance, particularly calcium deficit, can lead to tetany.

- The immediate goal of therapy is to control and decrease the inflammation of the pancreas.
- Volume replacement with fluids such as lactated Ringer's injection or normal human serum albumin is used to restore blood volume and prevent hypovolemic shock.

Endocrine and Metabolic

- Antibiotics are used to control microorganisms causing biliary pancreatitis and acute necrotizing pancreatitis.
- Opiates may be prescribed for pain relief.
- Nursing care centers on serial assessments, pain management, fluid replacement, nutrition and medication teaching, behavioral change toward alcohol abstinence.
- During the acute phase of pancreatitis, nurses should focus on continued monitoring and teaching.

Parathyroid Imbalance — Hyperparathyroidism and Hypoparathyroidism

Hyperparathyroidism is the clinical condition associated with oversecretion of parathyroid hormone (PTH). Primary hyperparathyroidism, the most common form, is a gland dysfunction that originates in the parathyroid gland. Secondary hyperparathyroidism, in contrast, is a parathyroid gland dysfunction that occurs in response to a disorder elsewhere in the body, such as chronic renal failure. The primary function of PTH is to regulate calcium and phosphorus balance by affecting gastrointestinal (GI) absorption of calcium, bone resorption (removal of bone tissue by absorption) of calcium, and renal regulation of both calcium and phosphorus.

Hypoparathyroidism is a rare clinical syndrome and is associated with a deficiency or absence of PTH or a decreased peripheral action of PTH. Although both hypocalcemia and hyperphosphatemia result from hypoparathyroidism, hypocalcemia accounts for the majority of clinical manifestations.

Where It Occurs

- Primary hyperparathyroidism affects women, especially postmenopausal and elderly women, more than men; is more frequent in individuals older than 50 years; and is unusual in children.
- Hypoparathyroidism may occur at any age, in both sexes, and in all races and ethnicities.

Signal Symptoms

- May be asymptomatic: hyperparathyroidism (hypercalcemia) symptoms include polyuria, anorexia, and constipation, as well as weakness, fatigue, drowsiness, decreased mental acuity, and lethargy.
- Hypoparathyroidism (hypocalcemia) symptoms include abdominal pain, nausea and vomiting, diarrhea, and anorexia.

BE SAFE! Hypocalcemia may lead to tetany and compromise of airway and breathing.

Diagnostic Tests

Test	What It Tells	Patient Problems/ Nursing Care
Serum calcium: total calcium, including free ionized calcium and calcium bound with protein or organic ions	Accumulation of calcium above normal levels in the extracellular fluid compartment for hyperparathyroidism; deficit in the same levels of calcium in hypoparathyroidism	Knowledge deficit: explain procedures. Patient will need venipuncture.
Serum PTH level	Determines presence of hypoparathyroidism	Knowledge deficit: explain procedures. Patient will need venipuncture.

Treatment and Nursing Care

Potential Nursing Diagnoses*

Activity intolerance
Ineffective airway clearance
Fatigue
Nausea
Risk for injury

▨ *BE SMART!* Assess patient's mobility and prevent risk of falls.

- Surgical removal of the parathyroid glands is the only definitive treatment and is the treatment of choice for primary hyperparathyroidism.
- Conjugated estrogen (Premarin) decreases the sensitivity of bones to increased PTH, thereby increasing bone calcium for the patient with hyperparathyroidism.
- Nurses should increase the hyperparathyroidism patient's mobility, protect the patient from injury, monitor for possible complications, and provide patient education.
- The treatment for hypoparathyroidism is to increase the ingestion and absorption of calcium either intravenously or by oral supplement.
- The primary nursing goal for hypoparathyroidism is the prevention of hypocalcemia in the high-risk population: patients with recent neck surgery.

Pituitary Tumor

Pituitary tumors are generally anterior lobe adenomas. Microadenomas are smaller than 1 cm, and macroadenomas are larger than 1 cm. Although microadenomas may cause complications because of over-produced pituitary hormones, they generally do not damage surrounding tissue. Because of their size, macroadenomas can be locally invasive, often damaging normal pituitary tissue and nearby nerves and parts of the brain. Most pituitary tumors are nonmalignant, but because of their invasiveness, they are considered neoplastic conditions.

Some 75% of pituitary adenomas are functional (hormone-producing) tumors. The hormone produced by an adenoma strongly influences its signs and symptoms and thus the choice of diagnostic tests and treatment. Adenomas are classified as prolactinomas, or prolactin-producing adenomas (30% of pituitary tumors); somatotrophin-secreting adenomas (15–20%); corticotrophin, or adrenocorticotropic hormone (ACTH)–secreting adenomas (10–15%); gonadotrophin-secreting adeno-mas (very small percentage); thyrotropin-secreting adenomas (very small percentage); null cell adenomas (15–20%); and plurihormonal (mixed-cell) adenomas. Pituitary tumors lead to hormone excess, hormone deficien-cies, or any combination of imbalances. In addition, as the tumor grows, it replaces normal pituitary gland tissue. Pituitary tumors seem to be genetic in origin.

Where It Occurs

- Approximately 70% of pituitary tumors occur in people between 30 and 50 years old.
- Twice as many females as males develop pituitary tumors.

Signal Symptoms

- Slowly developing and progressing symptoms: visual symptoms are the most common (blurred vision or double vision progressing to blindness, diplopia, ptosis); headache.
- Endocrine dysfunction: decreased sexual interest, menstrual irregularities, impotence, atrophy of breasts, testes.
- Anxiety, personality changes, seizure activity, and even dementia.
- Weakness, fatigue, sensitivity to cold, and constipation.
- Reduced muscle strength, obesity or weight loss depending on endocrine function.

BE SAFE! Although the tumors are generally benign, they must be removed because of the risk of impinging on vital structures.

Diagnostic Tests

Test	What It Tells	Patient Problems/ Nursing Care
Growth hormone	Functional (hormone-producing) tumor elevates levels of various hormones	Knowledge deficit: explain procedures. Patient will need venipuncture.
Gonadotrophins: follicle-stimulating hormone	Functional tumor elevates levels of various hormones	Knowledge deficit: explain procedures. Patient will need venipuncture.

Treatment and Nursing Care

Potential Nursing Diagnoses*

Disturbed sensory perception (visual)
Fatigue
Pain (acute)
Anxiety
Risk for injury

> **BE SMART!** Provide pre- and postoperative teaching to limit complications.

- The main treatment for many pituitary tumors is surgery, but medications may relieve symptoms and sometimes shrink the tumor.
- Prolactin inhibitors shrink prolactin-secreting tumors in 1 to 6 months.
- Reassure patient that treatment will manage symptoms.
- Nurses should focus on postoperative care and minimization of discomfort. Assess for neurological changes postoperatively and for signs of bleeding and infection.

Thyroid Imbalance—Hyperthyroidism, Hypothyroidism, and Thyrotoxicosis

Hyperthyroidism is a condition caused by excessive overproduction of thyroid hormone by the thyroid gland. The condition is a type of thyrotoxicosis, which is an elevation in the serum levels of thyroid hormones. The thyroid hormones (triiodothyronine [T3] and thyroxine [T4]), produced in the thyroid gland under the control of thyroid-stimulating hormone (TSH), regulate the body's metabolism. Sustained thyroid hormone overproduction causes a hypermetabolic state that affects most of the body organs, such as the heart, gastrointestinal tract, brain, muscles, eyes, and skin.

Hypothyroidism occurs when the thyroid gland produces a deficient amount of the thyroid hormones, resulting in a lowered basal metabolism.

Where It Occurs

- Hyperthyroidism is more frequently found in women than in men, is most typically diagnosed in 20- to 40-year-olds, and is slightly more common in white and Hispanic individuals than in African American individuals.
- Hypothyroidism is most frequently found in women between ages 30 and 50 years and may be higher in white females than in other races and ethnicities.

Signal Symptoms

- Hyperthyroidism: heat, excessive perspiration, and increased appetite; weight loss, abdominal cramping, frequent bowel movements; nervousness, irritability, restlessness, sleep disturbance.
- Hypothyroidism: cold intolerance, constipation, fatigue even with little activity, weight gain; aches and stiffness, generalized weakness, slowing of intellectual functions, impaired memory, loss of initiative.

BE SAFE! Deficits and excesses of thyroid hormone can lead to significant cardiopulmonary and neurological deficits and need prompt correction.

Diagnostic Tests

Test	What It Tells	Patient Problems/ Nursing Problems
TSH assay	Levels are either decreased (hypothyroidism) or increased (hyperthyroidism)	Knowledge deficit: explain procedures. Patient will need venipuncture.
T4 radioimmunoassay	Levels are decreased in hypothyroidism and increased in hyperthyroidism	Knowledge deficit: explain procedures. Patient will need venipuncture.

Treatment and Nursing Care

Potential Nursing Diagnoses*

Anxiety
Hyperthermia
Hypothermia
Activity intolerance
Fatigue

> **BE SMART!** Monitor the patient with hypothyroidism carefully for cardiac complications.

- Radioactive iodine is given to treat hyperthyroidism for two purposes: for diagnostic imaging in low doses and for therapeutic destruction of the thyroid gland in larger doses.
- Propylthiouracil (PTU) returns the patient with hyperthyroidism to the euthyroid (normal) state.
- Nursing interventions for hyperthyroidism center on ongoing monitoring, protecting the patient from injury, reducing stress, and initiating teaching.
- The treatment of choice for hypothyroidism is to provide thyroid hormone supplements to correct hormonal deficiencies.
- Levothyroxine sodium returns the patient to the euthyroid (normal) state.
- Nursing care for hypothyroidism focuses on monitoring patient intake and output and maximizing patient comfort.

Anaphylaxis

Anaphylactic shock, or anaphylaxis, is an immediate, life-threatening allergic reaction caused by a systemic antigen-antibody immune response to a foreign substance (antigen) introduced into the body. Anaphylaxis is caused by a type I, immunoglobulin E–mediated hypersensitivity reaction. The antigen combines with immunoglobulin E (IgE) on the surface of the mast cells and precipitates a release of histamine and other chemical mediators such as serotonin and slow-reacting substance of anaphylaxis (SRS-A). The resulting increased capillary permeability, smooth muscle contraction, and vasodilation account for the cardiovascular collapse. More than one organ system must be involved to be considered anaphylaxis, and those organs are most commonly the heart, lungs, skin, and gastrointestinal systems.

Anaphylaxis can result from a variety of causes, but it most commonly occurs in response to food, medications, and insect bites.

Where It Occurs

▪ Women appear to be slightly more susceptible than men to anaphylactic shock.
▪ Older people have a greater risk of anaphylaxis than younger people.

Signal Symptoms

▪ Rash, swelling, throat tightness, nausea, vomiting, tachycardia, headache, seizure, weakness, and lightheadedness.
▪ Symptoms typically begin within 5 to 30 minutes.

BE SAFE! Make sure the patient has a patent airway. A closed airway is a critical emergency.

Diagnostic Tests

No specific laboratory tests are required to diagnose anaphylactic shock, although diagnostic tests may be performed to rule out other causes of the symptoms, such as congestive heart failure, myocardial infarction, or status asthmaticus. If a patient is seen soon after the event, the following diagnostic tests may be helpful in confirming the diagnosis: plasma histamine, urinary histamine metabolites, or serum tryptase.

Treatment and Nursing Care

Potential Nursing Diagnoses*

Ineffective airway clearance
Impaired gas exchange
Knowledge deficit (medication and avoidance of allergen)
Impaired skin integrity

> **BE SMART!** Teach patient to carry an EpiPen (epinephrine) in case of emergency and to avoid the allergen.

- The plan of care depends on the severity of the reaction.
- Epinephrine decreases inflammation and allergic response.
- Diphenhydramine (Benadryl) may be given to inhibit further histamine release.
- The most important priority for nurses is to ensure adequacy of the airway, breathing, and circulation.
- Teach patient and family how to prevent future allergic reaction.

Aplastic Anemia

Aplastic, or hypoplastic, anemia is a bone marrow failure characterized by a decrease in all formed elements of peripheral blood and its bone marrow. If all elements are suppressed—resulting in loss of production of healthy erythrocytes, platelets, and granulocytes—the condition is known as pancytopenia. Onset is often insidious and may become chronic; however, onset may be rapid and overwhelming when the cause is a myelotoxin (a poison that damages the bone marrow).

With complete bone marrow suppression, leukocytic failure may result in fulminating infections, greatly reducing the chances for complete recovery. Less severe cases may have an acute transient course or a chronic course with ultimate recovery, although the platelet count may remain subnormal, thus requiring a lifetime of precautions against bleeding. Aplastic anemia may produce fatal bleeding or infection, however, especially if it is idiopathic or stems from chloramphenicol or infectious hepatitis.

Where It Occurs

■ Incidence of the condition is fairly low, without apparent sex or age preference.
■ Congenital hypoplastic anemia occurs in infants in the third month of life, and Fanconi's anemia occurs in children under age 10.

Signal Symptoms

■ Dyspnea, headache, intolerance for activity, progressive fatigue, malaise, chills and possibly fever, easy bruising, or frank bleeding.
■ Jaundiced or pale skin.

BE SAFE! Check for signs of increased bruising or bleeding.

Diagnostic Tests

Test	What It Tells	Patient Problems/ Nursing Care
Complete blood count	Red blood cells, white blood cells, and reticulocyte counts are all decreased by the condition as a result of injury to the stem cells	Knowledge deficit: explain procedures. Patient will need venipuncture.

Treatment and Nursing Care

Potential Nursing Diagnoses*

Risk for infection
Risk for injury
Impaired skin integrity
Knowledge deficit (medications, immunosuppression)

BE SMART! Protect the patient from infection after a bone marrow transplantation.

- If anemia is caused by a particular agent or drug, withdrawing it is usually the first step in treatment.
- Bone marrow transplantation is the treatment of choice for severe aplastic anemia.
- Corticosteroids stimulate erythroid production.
- Nurses should focus on limiting the chances of infection, teaching, and post-transplantation management.

Blood Transfusion Reaction

Blood transfusion reactions are adverse responses to the infusion of any blood component, including red cells, white cells, platelets, plasma, cryoprecipitate, or factors. They may be classified as acute (within 24 hours of administration) or delayed (occurring days, weeks, months, or even years later). They range from mild urticarial reactions that may be treated easily to fatal hemolytic reactions.

The immune system recognizes red blood cells, platelets, white blood cells, or immunoglobulins as "non-self" because the donor's blood carries foreign proteins that are incompatible with the recipient's antibodies. Typing, screening, and matching of blood units before administration eliminates most incompatibilities, but all potential incompatibilities cannot be screened out in the matching process.

Where It Occurs

- Infants and the elderly are more likely to experience problems of fluid overload with transfusion, and children are more likely to develop transfusion-related HIV infections than are adults.
- Nonhemolytic febrile reactions and extravascular hemolytic reactions are more common in females who have been pregnant.

Signal Symptoms

- Heat or pain at the site of transfusion, fever, chills, chest tightness, lower back pain, abdominal pain, nausea, difficulty breathing, itching, and a feeling of impending doom.
- Hives, changes in skin color, and edema.

BE SAFE! The most life-threatening complication is an impaired airway. Monitor airway patency if an allergic reaction is suspected.

Diagnostic Tests

Test	What It Tells	Patient Problems/ Nursing Care
Free hemoglobin: urine and plasma	Transfusion reaction leads to escape of hemoglobin from red blood cells during IV hemolysis	Knowledge deficit: explain all procedures. Patient may need a venipuncture.

Treatment and Nursing Care

Potential Nursing Diagnoses*

Risk for ineffective airway clearance
Hyperthermia
Impaired skin integrity
Pain (acute)

BE SMART! A change in vital signs from baseline may indicate the beginning of a transfusion reaction.

- Prevention is a crucial element in treating blood transfusion reactions.
- Epinephrine is given for severe reactions for its pressor effect and bronchodilation.
- Glucocorticoids are anti-inflammatory agents that limit laryngeal swelling.
- Nursing care should focus on attention to detail to prevent blood transfusion reactions by checking identification and frequent monitoring of vital signs.

Cytomegalovirus Infection

Cytomegalovirus (CMV) is a member of the herpes simplex virus group. The virus, transmitted by human contact, results in an infection so mild that it is usually overlooked because no symptoms are present.

Immunosuppressed patients, however, and particularly patients who have received transplanted organs, are highly susceptible to CMV. Generally, the CMV infection occurs 4 to 6 weeks after the implementation of increased doses of immunosuppressive drugs to treat rejection.

The virus generally inhabits the salivary glands in a latent infection that is reactivated by pregnancy, blood transfusions, or immunosuppressive medications. Benign in people with normal immune systems, the virus can be devastating to an unborn fetus or a person with immunosuppression. The virus is spread throughout the body by the white blood cells (lymphocytes and mononuclear cells) to organs such as the liver, lungs, gastrointestinal (GI) tract, and central nervous system (CNS), leading to cellular inflammation and possibly organ dysfunction. At least 60% of the U.S. population has been exposed to CMV.

Where It Occurs

- Fetuses and infants are at particular risk because intrauterine CMV infection is the most common congenital infection.
- CMV mononucleosis is the most common form of CMV infection, and it occurs at about 25 to 30 years of age.
- Men who have sex with men are a high-risk group with respect to CMV, as are people receiving immunosuppressive drugs such as those with rheumatoid arthritis, systemic lupus erythematosus, Crohn's disease, or psoriasis. Immunocompromised people can experience many inflammatory conditions such as pneumonia, hepatitis, myelitis, and colitis.

Signal Symptoms

- Many people have no symptoms from a CMV infection; others may have mild symptoms such as a fever of unknown origin and/or sore throat.
- Infants may show signs of delayed development, jaundice, petechial rash, respiratory distress, and hearing loss.
- Most severe signs and symptoms in adults occur with liver or CNS involvement (mental status changes, irritability, lethargy, seizures, and coma).

BE SAFE! Children's day-care environments may promote transmission both to children and from children to parents. The virus is transmitted by saliva and urine.

Diagnostic Tests

Test	What It Tells	Patient Problems/ Nursing Care
Antigen testing and polymerase chair reaction	Detects the presence of antigens against the virus or genetic material from the virus	Knowledge deficit: explain procedures. Patient will need venipuncture.
Culture of the urine, sputum, or mouth swab	Presence of virus confirms the diagnosis	Knowledge deficit: explain procedures. Avoid contamination of the specimen.

Treatment and Nursing Care

Potential Nursing Diagnoses*

Risk for infection (spread or reactivation)
Disturbed thought processes

BE SMART! Infants with congenital abnormalities require careful monitoring of growth and developmental patterns throughout infancy.

- Treatment focuses on preventing complications and relieving symptoms; treatment varies depending on the type and degree of infection.
- Ganciclovir inhibits DNA production in CMV and foscarnet inhibits replication of virus.
- To prevent transmission in children in day care, the following is important: wash hands well after changing diapers or feeding young children; do not share food, drink, utensils, or toothbrushes used by children; clean toys and countertops that come in contact with children's urine or saliva.
- Pregnant women who are exposed to CMV may have infants with CMV.
- Important nursing priorities are to maintain an adequate level of functioning, prevent complications, support the recuperative process, and provide information about the disease process, prognosis, and treatment.

Disseminated Intravascular Coagulation

Disseminated intravascular coagulation (DIC) is a life-threatening hemostatic disorder in which bleeding and clotting occur simultaneously. It is also called *consumptive coagulopathy* and *defibrination syndrome*. The pathophysiology involves an overactivation of the clotting mechanisms with both enhanced fibrin production leading to small clots and fibrinolysis leading to enhanced bleeding. As its name implies, tiny clots accumulate in the microcirculation (capillaries) throughout the body, depleting the blood supply of its clotting factors. These microemboli interfere with blood flow and lead to ischemia and organ damage. As the clots begin to lyse, fibrin degradation products (FDPs), which have an anticoagulant property of their own, are released. The FDPs, along with decreased levels of clotting factors in the bloodstream, lead to massive bleeding internally from the brain, kidneys, adrenals, heart, and other organs or from any wounds and old puncture sites.

Because DIC is somewhat difficult to diagnose, the following definition may be helpful in understanding the disorder: a systemic thrombohemorrhagic coagulation disorder associated with well-defined clinical situations and laboratory evidence of coagulant activation, fibrinolytic activation, inhibitor consumption, and biochemical evidence of end-organ damage. It is associated with a number of conditions such as sepsis, trauma and injury, transfusion reaction, solid tumors, liver failure, pregnancy and childbirth, and aneurysms.

Where It Occurs

- Women of childbearing age who develop pregnancy-induced hypertension and HELLP (hemolysis, elevated liver, low platelet) syndrome are potential candidates to develop DIC.
- Other high-risk patients are those with neoplasms (often the elderly), sepsis, or traumatic injuries (often young adult males) such as burns and crush injuries.
- Other than the association with childbirth, there are no sex and age factors associated with DIC.

Signal Symptoms

- Bleeding (wounds, vaginal), petechiae, ecchymoses, hematoma formation, epistaxis, hematuria, conjunctival hemorrhage, and hemoptysis.
- Severe joint, back pain, or muscle pain.

> **BE SAFE!** DIC can be rapidly progressing and life threatening if the coagulation disorder is not reversed promptly.

Diagnostic Tests

Test	What It Tells	Patient Problems/Nursing Care
Antithrombin III	Irreversible complexing of thrombin and circulating coagulation factors with antithrombin lower this level	Knowledge deficit: explain procedures. Patient will need venipuncture.
D-dimer	Elevated levels indicates DIC	Knowledge deficit: explain procedures. Patient will need venipuncture.

Treatment and Nursing Care

Potential Nursing Diagnoses*

Fluid volume deficit
Pain (acute)
Ineffective tissue perfusion (cerebral, peripheral)
Impaired tissue integrity

> **BE SMART!** Fluid volume resuscitation with colloids or crystalloids, or blood products is necessary in serious cases.

- Because DIC always occurs in association with another condition, medical treatment focuses on correcting the underlying disorder; in addition, the physician seeks to return the patient to normal hemostasis.

- Heparin inactivates thrombin and factors X and IX by antithrombin III.
- Antithrombin III replacement is used for moderately severe to severe DIC.
- Nurses should provide emotional support and educate the patient and family about the interventions and expected outcomes.

Hemophilia

Hemophilia refers to a group of congenital coagulation disorders characterized by a deficiency or malfunction of specific clotting factors. Hemophilia A, or classic hemophilia, is caused by a defect in factor VIII (antihemophilic factor). Hemophilia B, or Christmas disease, is less common and is caused by a defect in factor IX (plasma thromboplastin component, or Christmas factor). Hemophilia C, or factor XI (plasma thromboplastin antecedent) deficiency, is even more rare.

Persons with hemophilia can form a platelet plug but cannot form a stable clot. Clinical manifestations and complications of hemophilia are usually secondary to recurrent bleeding. All forms of hemophilia are the result of an X-linked recessive trait disorder.

Where It Occurs

- Hemophilia is an X-linked recessive condition. Therefore it occurs mostly in males.
- Rates of hemophilia for whites, African Americans, and Hispanic males in the United States are similar but lower for Asian Americans.

Signal Symptoms

- Bleeding disproportionate to the extent of a traumatic injury is characteristic of hemophilia; typically, intermittent oozing develops over several hours or days after the injury or procedure.
- Wound healing is often delayed.
- Signs of hemorrhage include orthostasis, epistaxis, hemoptysis; bleeding into joints, warmth and pain in joints; central nervous system: headache, stiff neck, irritability, vomiting; gastrointestinal: hematemesis, melena; genitourinary: hematuria.

BE SAFE! If a male infant has excessive bleeding at circumcision or excessive bruising occurs when the infant becomes ambulatory, suspect hemophilia.

Diagnostic Tests

Test	What It Tells	Patient Problems/ Nursing Care
Genetic testing	Identifies genetic alterations from normal	Knowledge deficit: explain procedures. Patient will need venipuncture or buccal swab.
Assay of factors VIII, IX, XI	Determines level of activity of essential factors needed for blood clotting, which is decreased in patients with hemophilia	Knowledge deficit: explain procedures. Patient will need venipuncture.

Treatment and Nursing Care

Potential Nursing Diagnoses*

Risk for injury
Fluid volume deficit
Knowledge deficit (medications, treatment options, genetic testing)
Fear
Disturbed body image

BE SMART! Comprehensive hemophilia centers maintain a multidisciplinary approach to evidence-based care.

- Factor replacement therapy and drug therapy may be used prophylactically or to control mild or major bleeding episodes.
- Desmopressin stimulates rapid release of von Willebrand factor into the blood.
- Ambulatory replacement therapy at home for bleeding episodes is used for most patients, and hospitalization is reserved for life-threatening bleeding episodes.

■ Patient education is critical for self-management of medications, physical activity guidelines, prevention of injury.

■ Nursing care focuses on precautionary measures undertaken to avoid trauma that may precipitate bleeding episodes.

HIV Disease

Acquired immunodeficiency syndrome (AIDS) is the final result of an infection with HIV, a retrovirus. Despite its name, AIDS is a disease rather than a *syndrome*, which refers to collections of symptoms that do not have an easily identifiable cause. This name was more appropriate in the early years of the AIDS epidemic, when health-care providers were aware only of the late stages of the disease and did not fully understand its mechanisms. The more current name for the condition is *HIV disease*, which refers to the pathogen that causes AIDS and encompasses all the phases of the disease, from infection to the deterioration of the immune system.

The early, acute phase in an immunocompetent person occurs with widespread viral production and seeding of lymph tissues. The symptoms are generally nonspecific, such as sore throat, myalgia, fever, weight loss, and fatigue; they occur 3 to 6 weeks after infection and resolve 2 to 4 weeks later. As the disease progresses, people may remain asymptomatic or may develop a persistent generalized lymphadenopathy. In either case, HIV replication occurs primarily in the lymphoid tissues. HIV infection of lymphocytes and other cells that bear specific protein markers leads to lymphopenia and impaired T and B cell function. When HIV infection becomes advanced, it often is called *AIDS*, which generally occurs when the CD4 count is below 200/mL. AIDS is characterized by the appearance of opportunistic infections such as lymphoma, candidiasis, cytomegalovirus disease, herpes simplex, and Kaposi sarcoma.

Where It Occurs

■ Blacks/African Americans bear a disproportionate burden of HIV disease compared with other populations.

■ Sixty-eight percent of women with newly diagnosed HIV disease are black/African American.

- The patient may describe neurological manifestations, including headache, lightheadedness, memory loss, word-finding difficulty, inability to concentrate, and mood swings.
- Populations at risk: men who have sex with men, males, young adults, female sex workers, IV drug users.

Signal Symptoms

- Night sweats, lymphadenopathy, fever, weight loss, fatigue, and rash.
- Gastrointestinal disturbances such as nausea, vomiting, diarrhea, and anorexia.

BE SAFE! Teach patients to always use protection during sexual intercourse.

Diagnostic Tests

Test	What It Tells	Patient Problems/ Nursing Care
Enzyme-linked immunosorbent assay (ELISA) and Western blot	Positive result for HIV antibodies	Knowledge deficit: explain procedures. Patient will need venipuncture.
T lymphocyte and B lymphocyte subsets; CD4 counts, CD4 percentages	B and T cell values decreased and CD4 counts less than 500/mL are generally associated with symptoms	Knowledge deficit: explain procedures. Patient will need venipuncture.

Treatment and Nursing Care

Potential Nursing Diagnoses*

Risk for infection
Ineffective sexuality patterns
Anxiety
Risk for compromised human dignity
Ineffective coping

BE SMART! To prevent transmission from mothers to babies, consider maternal testing, use antiviral therapy, consider Cesarean delivery, and avoid breastfeeding.

- Nucleoside analog reverse transcriptase inhibitors decrease HIV replication by incorporation into the strand of DNA, leading to chain termination.
- Nucleotide reverse transcriptase inhibitors also decrease HIV replication by incorporation into the strand of DNA, leading to chain termination.
- Supportive management consists of treatment of malignancies with chemotherapy and irradiation, treatment of infections as they develop, and management of discomfort with analgesia.
- Prophylaxis for *Pneumocystis jiroveci* with Bactrim may be necessary for immunosuppressed patients.
- During the more acute and severe stages of the illness, nursing interventions focus on maximizing the patient's health and promoting comfort.
- Teach patient about medications, lifestyle changes, physical activity, and sexual behaviors.

Hodgkin's Disease

Hodgkin's disease is a group of neoplastic disorders characterized by painless, progressive enlargement of the lymph nodes, spleen, and other lymphoid tissue. The enlargement is caused by a proliferation of lymphocytes, histiocytes, eosinophils, and Reed-Sternberg giant cells, the cells that characterize Hodgkin's disease; their presence classifies a lymphoma as Hodgkin's, and their absence classifies a lymphoma as non-Hodgkin's. Generally, the disease tends to begin within a single lymph node region and spreads to nodes in close proximity. Only late in the disease does widespread dissemination occur.

The cause of Hodgkin's disease is unknown, but genetics are linked and possibly Epstein-Barr virus (EBV).

Where It Occurs

- Hodgkin's disease tends to strike in young adulthood from the ages of 15 to 38 and is more common in men than in women.
- When children get the disease, approximately 85% of the patients are male.

- There is also a bimodal incidence, with the first major peak being in young adults and the second peak later in life after age 50.
- Hodgkin's disease is more common among whites than among Asian Americans and African Americans.

Signal Symptoms

- Early: peripheral adenopathy (cervical, supraclavicular, and mediastinal).
- Fever, night sweats, and recent weight loss.
- Cough, chest pain, shortness of breath, pruritus, back or bone pain.

BE SAFE! Hodgkin's lymphoma is considered to be a curable malignancy and should be diagnosed promptly.

Diagnostic Tests

Test	What It Tells	Patient Problems/ Nursing Care
Lymph node biopsy or bone marrow biopsy	Determines extent of disease and allows for staging of disease	Knowledge deficit: explain procedures. Check for bleeding and infection.
Computed tomography (CT) scan or magnetic resonance imaging (MRI) of chest, abdomen, and pelvis	Assists with staging	Knowledge deficit: explain procedures.

Treatment and Nursing Care

Potential Nursing Diagnoses*

Risk for infection
Pain (acute)
Ineffective breathing pattern
Ineffective coping
Anxiety

BE SMART! Discuss treatment options with the patient and answer all questions.

- Treatment begins with accurate classification and staging.
- In general, radiation is used for early, less extensive disease, whereas a combination of radiation and chemotherapy or chemotherapy and other drugs are used for more advanced disease.
- If the disease does not respond to standard treatment, bone marrow transplantation may be offered, either as part of a clinical trial or outside of a clinical trial.
- The primary nursing roles are to maintain comfort, protect the patient from infection, provide teaching and support about the complications of the treatment, and give emotional support.

Idiopathic Thrombocytopenia Purpura

Idiopathic thrombocytopenic purpura (ITP) is an acquired hemorrhagic disorder characterized by an increased destruction of platelets because of antiplatelet antibodies. The antibodies attach to the platelets, reduce their life span, and lead to a platelet count below 100,000/mm^3 but occasionally as low as 5,000/mm^3. ITP can be acute or chronic. Acute ITP is generally a self-limiting childhood disorder, whereas chronic ITP predominantly affects adults and is characterized by thrombocytopenia of more than 6 months.

The most life-threatening complication of ITP is intracerebral hemorrhage, which is most likely to occur if the platelet count falls below 1,000/mm^3. Hemorrhage into the kidneys, abdominal cavity, or retroperitoneal space is also possible. Acute ITP is thought to be a response to a viral infection, whereas chronic ITP generally has no underlying viral association and is often linked to immunological disorders.

Where It Occurs

- Acute ITP affects children of both sexes between ages 2 and 9 years.
- Chronic ITP occurs mainly between ages 20 and 50 years and affects women almost three times as often as men.

Signal Symptoms

- Because the symptoms of chronic ITP are usually insidious, patients may not have noticed an increase in symptoms.
- Diffuse petechiae (red to purple dots on the skin, 1–3 mm in size), epistaxis, or bruises on the skin and in the oral mucosa, bleeding gums.
- In both types of ITP, the spleen and liver are often slightly palpable, with lymph node swelling.

BE SAFE! For young children, help the parent create a safe environment that will prevent falls, and cover any sharp objects that might lead to injury and bleeding.

Diagnostic Tests

Test	What It Tells	Patient Problems/ Nursing Care
Platelet count	Platelets are consumed during clot formation, and the degree of platelet suppression predicts the severity of symptoms	Knowledge deficit: explain procedures. Patient will need venipuncture.

Treatment and Nursing Care

Potential Nursing Diagnoses*

Risk for injury
Knowledge deficit (cause, complications, medications)
Disturbed body image
Impaired tissue integrity

BE SMART! Encourage patient or parents to avoid all medications that reduce platelets or platelet function, such as aspirin and NSAIDs.

- Treatment for ITP is primarily pharmacologic. Intravenous immune globulin increases antibody titer and antigen-antibody reaction.
- Glucocorticoids decrease inflammatory response.

- Splenectomy is reserved for the most critical cases when medical therapy has failed.
- Nursing care centers on instituting safety precautions to prevent injury and the resultant bleeding. Fall prevention is particularly important in young children and the elderly.

Iron Deficiency Anemia

Iron deficiency anemia (IDA), the most common form of anemia, is a condition in which normal body stores of iron and hemoglobin levels are decreased. IDA is caused by inadequate intake of iron, inadequate storage of iron, excessive loss of iron, or some combination of these conditions. The red blood cells (RBCs), which become pale (hypochromic) and small (microcytic), have a decreased ability to transport oxygen in sufficient quantities to meet body needs. Anemia is a decrease in circulating RBC mass; the usual criteria for anemia are hemoglobin of less than 12 g/dL with a hematocrit less than 36% in women and hemoglobin less than 14 g/dL with a hematocrit less than 41% in men.

The most common causes of IDA are menstrual blood loss and the increased iron requirements of pregnancy. Other causes include pica, hemorrhage, achlorhydria, surgical removal of the bowel, and genetic abnormalities.

Where It Occurs

- Young women, in particular, are at risk as a result of heavy menses or unwise weight-reduction plans, and in the United States, females have a higher incidence of IDA than do males.
- Women at highest risk for IDA are minority women who live in urban poverty.

Signal Symptoms

- Recent weight loss, fatigue, weakness, activity intolerance, dizziness, irritability, inability to concentrate, sensitivity to cold, heartburn, loss of appetite, diarrhea, or flatulence.
- Signs of inflammation (stomatitis) or eroded, tender, and swollen corners (angular stomatitis) of the mouth.

BE SAFE! Keep the patient safe from falls and injury until replacement therapy has resolved the activity intolerance and weakness.

Diagnostic Tests

Test	What It Tells	Patient Problems/ Nursing Care
Bone marrow biopsy	Cells show absent staining for iron	Pain (acute). Medicate if pain at the site persists. Risk for infection: Inspect puncture site.
Complete blood count	Blood count is decreased because cells are iron deficient	Knowledge deficit: explain procedures. Patient will need venipuncture.

Treatment and Nursing Care

Potential Nursing Diagnoses*

Activity intolerance
Fluid volume deficit
Imbalanced nutrition, less than body requirements
Risk for infection

BE SMART! Pregnant women may need iron supplements during the last half of pregnancy.

- The two primary goals of treatment are to diagnose and correct the underlying cause of the iron deficiency and to correct the iron deficit.
- Supplemental iron increases iron stores.
- Nursing interventions focus on preventing infections, promoting comfort, and teaching the patient.
- Usually activity restriction is unnecessary unless the patient has underlying cardiopulmonary disease.

Leukemia

Leukemia is a malignant disease of the blood-forming organs that leads to a transformation of stem cells or early committed precursor cells and thus to an abnormal overproduction of certain leukocytes. Two types of chronic leukemia commonly occur: chronic lymphocytic leukemia (CLL) and chronic myelogenous leukemia (CML). CLL involves lymphocytes (B cells), which derive from stem cells and circulate among blood, lymph nodes, and lymphatic organs. In CLL, an uncontrollable spread of abnormal, small lymphocytes occurs in the bone marrow, lymphoid tissues, and blood. In CLL, an underproduction of immunoglobulins (antibodies) leads to increased susceptibility to infections. Some patients also develop antibodies to red blood cells (RBCs) and platelets, which then leads to anemia and thrombocytopenia. CML is characterized by the abnormal overgrowth of myeloblasts, promyelocytes, metamyelocytes, and myelocytes (all granulocytic precursors) in body tissues, peripheral blood, and bone marrow. In CML, the bone marrow becomes 100% cellular (rather than 50% cellular and 50% fat, the normal composition). The spleen enlarges with a greatly expanded red pulp area. CML has two phases: insidious chronic phase and acute phase. In the insidious chronic phase, chronic leukemia originates in the pluripotent stem cell and shows an initial finding of hypercellular marrow with a majority of normal cells. After a relatively slow course for a median of 4 years, chronic leukemia invariably enters a blast crisis, or acute phase.

Acute leukemia results when white blood cell (WBC) precursors proliferate in the bone marrow and lymphatic tissues. The cells eventually spread to the peripheral blood and all body tissues. Leukemia is considered acute when it has a rapid onset and progression. There are two major forms of acute leukemia: lymphocytic leukemia and nonlymphocytic leukemia. Lymphocytic leukemia involves the lymphocytes (cells derived from the stem cells and that circulate among the blood, lymph nodes, and lymphatic organs) and lymphoid organs; nonlymphocytic leukemia involves hematopoietic stem cells that differentiate into monocytes, granulocytes, RBCs, and platelets. Acute myelogenous leukemia (AML) (also known as acute nonlymphocytic leukemia, or ANLL) causes the rapid accumulation of megakaryocytes (precursors to platelets), monocytes, granulocytes, and RBCs.

Where It Occurs

- Chronic leukemia affects mostly older adults, over age 50 years.
- Twice as many males as females develop chronic leukemia.
- CLL is rare in Asian countries, and in the United States, the incidence of CLL is also higher in whites than in African Americans.
- The majority of patients with acute lymphoblastic leukemia (ALL) are under 10 years of age, with the peak age for children to develop ALL between 2 and 3 years of age.
- AML tends to increase in occurrence in the teen years but most often strikes older people; the average age of a patient with AML is 65.
- Males are more susceptible to AML than are females, and the disease is more common in European Americans than in other Americans; more than twice as many European Americans as African Americans develop ALL.

Signal Symptoms

- Symptoms of chronic leukemia are nonspecific and vague. In CML, sometimes the first symptom is a dragging sensation caused by extreme splenomegaly, or it may be left upper quadrant pain caused by a splenic infarct. In CLL, swollen lymph nodes or enlarged liver and spleen may cause discomfort.
- Fever, chills, cutaneous bleeding, petechiae, tiredness, fatigue, anemia.
- Symptoms of acute leukemia are sudden onset of high fever and signs of abnormal bleeding (increased bruising, bleeding after minor trauma, nosebleeds, bleeding gums, petechiae, and prolonged menses). Patients may report fatigue and malaise, weight loss, palpitations, night sweats, and chills.

BE SAFE! Protect the patient from exposure to infection; encourage hand washing and ask family members with infections to stay away during hospitalizations.

Diagnostic Tests

Test	What It Tells	Patient Problems/ Nursing Care
Complete blood count and differential	Overproduction of WBCs halts production of RBCs and platelets	Knowledge deficit: explain procedures. Patient will need venipuncture.
Bone marrow aspiration/bone marrow biopsy	Biopsy reveals presence of leukemic blast phase cells and leukemic surface markers on cells	Pain (acute). Medicate if pain at the site persists. Risk for infection: Inspect puncture site.

Treatment and Nursing Care

Potential Nursing Diagnoses*

Risk for infection
Activity intolerance
Fatigue
Anxiety

> **BE SMART!** Discuss treatment options with the patient and family so that they are knowledgeable about all decisions.

- In CLL, because treatments destroy normal cells along with malignant ones, therapy focuses on the prevention and resolution of complications from induced pancytopenia (anemia, bleeding, and infection in particular).
- Therapy in the chronic phase of CML focuses on achieving (1) hematologic remission, (2) cytogenetic remission, and (3) molecular remission.
- Prednisone decreases autoimmune response.
- Chemotherapy controls CLL symptoms and prevents proliferation of WBCs.
- Nursing management for chronic leukemia focuses on providing comfort, support, and patient education and managing complications.
- The treatment for acute leukemia occurs in four phases: induction, consolidation, continuation, and treatment of (CNS) leukemia.

- Chemotherapeutic agents decrease replication of leukemia cells and kill them.
- Nursing care for acute leukemia focuses on teaching the patient and significant others about the course of the disease, the treatment options, and how to recognize complications.

Lupus Erythematosus

Lupus erythematosus is an autoimmune disease that affects the connective tissue of the body. The course of disease is variable and unpredictable, with episodes of remission and relapse. Lupus takes two forms. Systemic lupus erythematosus (SLE) is a multisystem inflammatory disease that affects any body system but primarily the musculoskeletal, cutaneous, renal, nervous, and cardiovascular systems. Discoid lupus erythematosus (DLE) is a less serious form of the disease that primarily affects the skin. DLE is characterized by skin lesions of the face, scalp, and ears. Longstanding lesions can cause scarring, hypopigmentation, and redness. Only 5% to 10% of patients with DLE develop SLE. The multisystem nature of SLE places the patient at risk for multiple complications, and the disease is ultimately fatal.

The cause of lupus erythematosus is not known, but it is thought to occur because of genetic, racial, hormonal, and environmental factors.

Where It Occurs

- SLE occurs most frequently in females between the ages of 15 and 45, with the average age of onset at 30 years.
- SLE affects women at least four times more frequently than men and, during childbearing years, up to 15 times more often than men.
- It is also more prominent in Asians and African Americans than it is in whites.
- DLE is more common in women than in men, and approximately 60% of cases are female patients in their late 20s or older.

Signal Symptoms

■ Fatigue, malaise, weight loss, anorexia, and fever.
■ Joint and muscle pain, puffiness of hands and feet, joint swelling and tenderness, hand deformities, and skin lesions such as the characteristic "butterfly rash" (fixed reddish and flat rash that extends over both cheeks and the bridge of the nose), maculopapular rash (small, colored area with raised red pimples), sensitivity to the sun, photophobia, vascular skin lesions, leg ulcers, oral ulcers, and hair loss.

BE SAFE! Encourage patients to avoid sun exposure, which might worsen skin lesions.

Diagnostic Tests

Diagnostic tests include complete blood count, antinuclear antibody, urinalysis, anti-DNA antibody, complement levels, anti–double-stranded DNA antibody assay, blood urea nitrogen, creatinine, and creatinine clearance. To be diagnosed with lupus, the patient must have at least four of the following criteria: malar rash, discoid rash, photosensitivity, oral ulcers, arthritis, serositis, renal disorders, neurological disorders, hematological disorders, immunological disorders, antinuclear antibody.

Treatment and Nursing Care

Potential Nursing Diagnoses*

Impaired skin integrity
Fatigue
Pain (acute)
Risk for infection
Activity intolerance

BE SMART! Patients need to maintain patterns of wellness, reduce stress, and maintain physical activity.

■ General supportive therapy includes adequate sleep and avoidance of fatigue because mild disease exacerbations may subside after several days of bedrest, but much of the therapy is pharmacologic.

- Corticosteroids control SLE in most severe or life-threatening cases (glomerulonephritis, debilitation from symptoms).
- Choline magnesium trisalicylate manages the inflammatory process.
- Nursing care includes helping the patient to manage pain and discomfort, make lifestyle changes, manage medications, and learn how to protect skin.

Multiple Myeloma

Multiple myeloma, also known as *plasma cell myeloma*, *malignant plasmacytoma*, and *myelomatosis*, is a type of cancer formed by malignant plasma cells. When a B lymphocyte is stimulated by a T cell, it develops into a mature, antibody-producing factory called a *plasma cell*. Multiple myeloma results from a transformed plasma cell that multiplies and produces antibody unceasingly, without stimulation. When plasma cells grow out of control, they generate tumors that infiltrate the bone marrow and other sites. Although multiple myeloma could be considered a lymphoma, it is generally classified differently and discussed separately because it presents a different profile of onset, symptoms, treatment, and prognosis.

The disease infiltrates bone and produces osteolytic lesions throughout the skeleton, destroying bones. In later stages, multiple myeloma infiltrates the body organs and destroys them as well. About 3 to 20 years of plasma cell growth may pass before symptoms become apparent. When patients do report symptoms, the disease is well advanced. The cause is unknown.

Where It Occurs

- Multiple myeloma is primarily a disease of late-middle-aged to elderly persons; the average age at diagnosis is 70 years, and it is rare before age 40.
- More men than women are affected.
- For unknown reasons, rates for African Americans are twice those for whites.

Signal Symptoms

■ Constant back pain that intensifies with exercise, other aching
bone pain, or arthritic-type joint pain.
■ Numbness, prickling, or tingling of the extremities (peripheral
paresthesia); confusion; fatigue; or weakness.
■ Pathological fractures, weakness, fatigue, activity intolerance.

BE SAFE! Use caution when moving patient or turning or positioning
to prevent pathological fractures.

Diagnostic Tests

Test	What It Tells	Patient Problems/ Nursing Care
Serum protein electrophoresis; urine protein electrophoresis	Identifies abnormal proteins produced by cancerous plasma cells as compared with product of normal plasma cells	Knowledge deficit: explain procedures. Patient will need venipuncture.
Bone marrow aspiration; bone marrow biopsy	Biopsy indicates plasma cell tumor	Pain (acute). Medicate if pain at the site persists.

Treatment and Nursing Care

Potential Nursing Diagnoses*

Pain (acute or chronic)
Risk for infection
Activity intolerance
Fatigue
Fluid volume deficit

BE SMART! Assess for signs of hypercalcemia: confusion, sleepiness,
fatigue, constipation, nausea, and thirst.

- Treatment depends on disease staging and generally consists of chemotherapy, radiation, prednisone, and as much ambulation as the patient can tolerate.
- Chemotherapy suppresses plasma cell growth and controls pain.
- Opioids and NSAIDs manage severe bone pain.
- Nursing interventions include educating the patient about the disease process and treatments and minimizing pain and discomfort.

Polycythemia

Polycythemia generically refers to an increased concentration of red blood cells (RBCs, or erythrocytes). This blood disorder has several causes and can be classified as primary, secondary, or relative polycythemia. Primary polycythemia (polycythemia vera) is a chronic, proliferative bone marrow disorder that leads to overproduction of RBCs, white blood cells (WBCs), and platelets and results in increased blood viscosity and platelet dysfunction. Secondary polycythemia causes excessive production of RBCs because of hypoxemia or tumors and is often triggered by overproduction of erythropoietin. Lastly, relative polycythemia is caused by reduced plasma volume. The RBC count is normal or even reduced, but increased blood concentration occurs because of increased concentration of cells compared with plasma.

Most complications of all types of polycythemia occur as a result of increased blood viscosity (hyperviscosity) or sudden blood loss (hemorrhage). Hyperviscosity may lead to thromboembolic events, such as organ thromboses or splenomegaly. Hemorrhage in any system can occur from platelet dysfunction. Hemorrhage and vasculitis may occur together because an excessive number of RBCs exert pressure on capillary walls.

Where It Occurs

- The incidence of primary polycythemia is the highest in middle-aged and older European American men, with a median onset age of 60.
- Condition has a genetic basis.

Signal Symptoms

- Headache, dizziness, hypoxemia.
- Ringing in the ears, visual changes.
- Pain (chest pain, intermittent claudications).
- Bleeding gums, epistaxis, increased bruising, gastrointestinal bleeding.
- Thromboembolism, enlarged spleen, itching.

BE SAFE! Manage pain and signs of hypoxemia rapidly with oxygen administration and rest.

Diagnostic Tests

Test	What It Tells	Patient Problems/ Nursing Care
Bone marrow biopsy	Biopsy reveals hypercellular bone marrow with residual fat, increased erythroid progenitors, increased maturing granulocytic precursors and megakaryocytes	Pain (acute): medicate if pain at the site persists.
Complete blood count	Reveals increased proliferation and production of bone marrow elements	Knowledge deficit: explain procedures. Patient will need venipuncture.

Treatment and Nursing Care

Potential Nursing Diagnoses*

Ineffective protection
Pain (acute)
Anxiety
Impaired tissue integrity

BE SMART! Many patients with polycythemia have a history of cardiac and pulmonary disease, particularly emphysema.

- In primary polycythemia, the treatment goal is to reduce blood viscosity.
- In secondary polycythemia, the treatment goal is to treat the disease that acts as a hypoxic trigger or causes increased production of erythropoietin.
- In relative polycythemia, the treatment goal is to prevent dehydration and thromboembolic conditions and to correct fluid volume deficits.
- Warfarin sodium (Coumadin) assists in preventing clot formation.
- The patient's activity level is a primary nursing concern.

Progressive Systemic Sclerosis

Progressive systemic sclerosis (SSc; scleroderma) is a rare, total body condition of the connective tissues in which skin hardening and thickening occurs along with tissue fibrosis and chronic inflammatory infiltration of multiple visceral organs. Characteristics of systemic sclerosis result from collagen deposition and fibrosis in tissues and organs. Alterations include vasomotor disturbances, skin changes, fibrosis of the subcutaneous tissue and muscles, and changes in the gastrointestinal system, lungs, heart, kidney, joints, and brain function.

These changes are thought to be autoimmune in nature with genetics, environmental, vascular, and circulatory factors involved. Patients with SSc may have increased risk of some cancers, particularly breast cancer.

Where It Occurs

- Women are four to nine times more likely than men to suffer from progressive systemic sclerosis.
- Individuals ages 30 to 50 years are most likely to develop the disease, whereas men in their 50s are most likely to show signs.

Signal Symptoms

■ Tightening of skin, itching, thickening of skin, edema and induration of skin, hyperpigmentation, whitening of the hands during cold exposure (vasomotor disturbance).

■ Difficulty swallowing, nausea, vomiting, weight loss, bloating, gastric reflux, diarrhea, fecal incontinence.

■ Shortness of breath on exertion, palpitations, chest pain, fatigue, weakness.

BE SAFE! Make sure that impaired swallowing is treated early so that the patient does not develop aspiration pneumonia.

Diagnostic Tests

Test	What It Tells	Patient Problems/ Nursing Care
Erythrocyte sedimentation rate (ESR)	Elevated due to inflammatory processes	Knowledge deficit: explain procedures. Patient will need venipuncture.

Treatment and Nursing Care

Potential Nursing Diagnoses*

Impaired skin integrity
Impaired swallowing
Diarrhea
Risk for injury
Disturbed body image

BE SMART! Encourage patients to stop smoking, which worsens condition.

■ Encourage patients to avoid exposure to cold temperature and to dress warmly during winter months.

■ Anti-inflammatory agents such as corticosteroids may be used.

- Calcium channel blockers, vasodilating drugs, prostacyclin analogs, or aspirin may be used to treat the condition. Make sure patient understands all medications.
- Other medications, depending on organ system involvement, might include angiotensin II inhibitors, proton pump inhibitors, and H_2 blockers, which can help to control reflux symptoms.
- Teach patient about medications, lifestyle changes, skin care, and strategies to stop smoking.

Rheumatoid Arthritis

Rheumatoid arthritis (RA) is a chronic, progressive, systemic disease characterized by recurrent inflammation of connective tissue, primarily diarthrodial joints (hinged joints that contain a cavity within the capsule that separates the bony elements to allow freedom of movement) and their related structures. The disease generally begins with inflammation of the synovial membrane, which becomes thickened and edematous. The thickened synovium, or pannus, erodes the articular cartilage and underlying bone, causing joint destruction. The small peripheral joints of the hand and wrist and the joints of the knees, ankles, elbows, and shoulders are usually affected symmetrically. The cervical spine may also be affected. Extra-articular involvement of the disease includes inflammation of the tendon sheaths; the bursae; and the connective tissue of the heart, lungs, pleurae, and arteries.

If the disease is left untreated, the inflammatory process of RA moves through four stages. In the first stage, synovitis is caused by congestion and edema of the synovial membrane and joint capsule. In the second stage, the formation of pannus, thickened layers of granulation tissue that cover and invade cartilage, begins and leads to eventual destruction of the joint capsule and bone. In the third stage, fibrous ankylosis is noted in the inflammatory process; this is the fibrous invasion of the pannus and scar formation that occludes joint space. In the fourth and final stage, the fibrous tissue calcifies, causing ankylosis and total immobility. Although the specific cause of RA is unknown, there is speculation about multiple causation, which includes infection, autoimmunity, and genetic factors and also environmental and hormonal factors.

Where It Occurs

- RA is two to three times more common in women than in men.
- The disease can occur at any age, although the onset peaks between 30 and 60 years of age.
- The main environmental risk is cigarette smoking.

Signal Symptoms

- Early: joint pain and swelling, fatigue, malaise, low-grade fever, weight loss, anemia, and anorexia.
- Late: joint problems such as deformities, contractures, immobility, and inability to perform the activities of daily living.

BE SAFE! Initiate treatment rapidly so that joint deterioration does not progress.

Diagnostic Tests

Test	What It Tells	Patient Problems/Nursing Care
Rheumatoid factor (Rose Waaler) and anticyclic citrullinated peptide antibody (anti-CCP) assay	Identifies unusual immunoglobulin G and M antibodies that develop against connective tissue disease	Knowledge deficit: explain procedures. Patient will need venipuncture.
Antinuclear antibody	Identifies antibodies to the body's own DNA and nuclear material	Knowledge deficit: explain procedures. Patient will need venipuncture.

Treatment and Nursing Care

Potential Nursing Diagnoses*

Pain (acute and chronic)
Impaired physical mobility
Activity intolerance

Fatigue
Ineffective role performance

- The goals of treatment are to relieve pain, inhibit the inflammatory response, preserve joint function, and prevent deformity.
- NSAIDs are used to relieve pain.
- Rest and stress reduction are important strategies to reduce exacerbations.
- Disease modifying antirheumatic drugs (DMARDs) slow disease progression and joint destruction.
- Prednisone reduces inflammation in people who do not respond to NSAIDs.
- Nursing care focuses on patient education in order to minimize discomfort and maximize independence.

Rocky Mountain Spotted Fever

Rocky Mountain spotted fever is a tick-borne disease found in all 48 contiguous United States. A small, intracellular parasite, *Rickettsia rickettsii*, is released from the salivary glands of some adult ticks. After exposure, the incubation period is usually about a week, but in cases of severe infection, it can be as short as 2 days. Complications, although uncommon, include pneumonia, pneumonitis, middle-ear infections, and parotitis. If the infection is left untreated, the associated rash may lead to peeling skin and even gangrene of the elbows, fingers, and toes. Life-threatening complications—such as disseminated intravascular coagulation, shock, and acute renal failure—occur rarely.

Where It Occurs

- Most reports indicate that the majority of those infected are male (60%) and under the age of 20 years (50%), although another peak in incidence occurs in men 60 to 69 years of age.
- Whites have twice the incidence that African Americans do.

Signal Symptoms

- Classic triad of symptoms: fever, rash, and a history of exposure to ticks.
- Fever, severe headache, joint pain, muscle and bone pain, malaise, and lethargy.
- Petechial rash, anorexia, nausea, vomiting, diarrhea, and abdominal pain.
- Acute infections may lead to serious complications: hypotension, dyspnea, shortness of breath.

BE SAFE! The infection needs to be treated rapidly with antibiotics.

Diagnostic Tests

Most often, the diagnosis of Rocky Mountain spotted fever is made as a result of clinical findings because diagnostic titers of antibodies are only detectable 10 days after the onset of illness. Other tests may include complement fixation titer, indirect hemagglutination titer, indirect immunofluorescence titer, and latex agglutination. Complete blood count may show thrombocytopenia (50% of patients) and anemia (30% of patients). Electrolytes may show hyponatremia (60% of patients).

Treatment and Nursing Care

Potential Nursing Diagnoses*

Risk for infection
Hyperthermia
Impaired skin integrity
Pain (acute)
Anxiety

BE SMART! Ask the patient about recent outdoor activities during the assessment phase.

- If the patient is critically ill, intubation, fluid resuscitation, and support of airway, breathing, and circulation are necessary.
- Antibiotics are used to kill the microorganism and fight infection.
- Tick removal may be necessary.
- Nursing care focuses on increasing comfort, monitoring for complications, and educating the patient.

Sickle Cell Anemia

Sickle cell disease (SCD) is a genetic, autosomal recessive disorder that results in abnormalities of the globin genes of the hemoglobin (Hb) molecule of the red blood cells (RBCs). Sickle cell anemia, the severest of the sickle cell disorders, is homozygous and has no known cure. Sickle cell trait occurs when a child inherits normal Hb from one parent and Hb S (the abnormal Hb) from the other; people with the sickle cell trait are carriers only and rarely manifest the clinical signs of the disorder.

The RBCs that contain more Hb S than Hb A are prone to sickling when they are exposed to decreased oxygen tension in the blood. The cells become more elongated, thus the term *sickle*. Once sickled, RBCs are more rigid, fragile, and rapidly destroyed. The RBCs therefore have a short survival time (30–40 days, as compared with a normal 120-day survival rate), a decreased oxygen-carrying capacity, and low Hb content. They cannot flow easily through tiny capillary beds and may become clumped and cause obstructions. The obstructions can lead to ischemia and necrosis, which produce the major clinical manifestations of pain. Two factors, hypoxemia and a change in the condition of the blood, have been identified as producing sickling, although the exact cause is unknown.

Where It Occurs

- Sickle cell occurs most frequently in African Americans but also occurs in African, Mediterranean, Caribbean, Middle Eastern, and Central American populations.
- Clinical symptoms rarely appear before the child is 6 months old and occur in both boys and girls.

Signal Symptoms

- The extent of the symptoms depends on the amount of Hb S that is present.
- Similar to the other types of hemolytic anemia: malaise, fever, fatigue, pallor, jaundice, and irritability.

■ Vaso-occlusive crisis: acute and sudden pain in the abdomen, bones, joints, and soft tissue; dactylitis (bilateral painful and swollen hands or feet), acute joint necrosis, or acute abdomen; organ infarctions and infection; kidney papillary necrosis leading to dilute urine; abdominal distention and pain.

> **BE SAFE!** Patients with vaso-occlusive crisis need significant amounts of pain medication for relief.

Diagnostic Tests

Test	What It Tells	Patient Problems/ Nursing Care
Genetic testing	Identifies expressed mutations in single genes	Knowledge deficit: explain procedures. Patient will need venipuncture.
Peripheral blood smear	RBCs have a characteristic sickle shape caused by structurally abnormal Hb molecules	Knowledge deficit: explain procedures. Patient will need venipuncture.

Treatment and Nursing Care

Potential Nursing Diagnoses*

Delayed growth and development
Pain (acute)
Social isolation
Fatigue
Impaired physical mobility

> **BE SMART!** Teach the patient about medications and lifestyle changes to reduce the potential of exacerbations.

■ Although SCD cannot be cured, there are many treatment alternatives to prevent exacerbations, limit complications, and manage sickle cell crises.

■ Hydroxyurea (Hydrea) increases total and fetal hemoglobin in children, thereby reducing sickling, white blood cell accumulation, and symptoms of vaso-occlusion.

- Analgesia relieves pain. Patients may need transfusions for episodes of acute pain or anemia.
- Educate patients to recognize infection anemia. Infections should be treated early and promptly.
- Nurses should stress the importance of maintaining hydration and assist with pain management in the case of an acute crisis.

Calcium Imbalance—Hypercalcemia and Hypocalcemia

Hypercalcemia occurs with a serum calcium level above 10.5 mg/dL in the bloodstream, although clinical manifestations generally occur at concentrations exceeding 12 mg/dL. It develops when an influx of calcium into the circulation overwhelms the calcium regulatory hormones (parathyroid hormone [PTH] and metabolites of vitamin D) and renal calciuric mechanisms or when there is a primary abnormality of one or both of these hormones. At levels above 13 mg/dL, renal failure and soft tissue calcification may occur. Hypercalcemic crisis exists when the serum level reaches 15 mg/dL. Serious cardiac dysrhythmias and hypokalemia can result as the body wastes potassium in preference to calcium. Hypercalcemia at this level can cause coma and cardiac arrest. It is considered to be a serious electrolyte imbalance. More than 90% of cases of hypercalcemia result from primary hyperparathyroidism or malignancy.

Hypocalcemia is a diminished calcium level, below 8.5 mg/dL, in the bloodstream, and is a more common clinical problem than hypercalcemia. When calcium levels drop, neuromuscular excitability occurs in smooth, skeletal, and cardiac muscle, causing the muscles to twitch. The result can lead to cardiac dysrhythmias. Hypocalcemia can also cause increased capillary permeability, pathological fractures, and decreased blood coagulation. Most severe cases result in tetany (condition of prolonged, painful spasms of the voluntary muscles of the fingers and toes [carpopedal spasm] as well as the facial muscles), which, if left untreated, leads to carpopedal and laryngeal spasm, seizures, and respiratory arrest. The most frequent cause of hypocalcemia is a low albumin level.

Where It Occurs

■ Hypercalcemia can occur in any age group, in both sexes, and in all races and ethnicities.

■ Hypocalcemia can occur at any age, in both sexes, and in all races and ethnicities, but infants, children, and the elderly are at high risk.

Signal Symptoms

- Hypercalcemia: anorexia, nausea, vomiting, constipation, polyuria, or polydipsia; may cause personality changes.
- Hypocalcemia: anxiety, irritability, twitching around the mouth, laryngospasm, and convulsions.
- Hypocalcemia: tingling or numbness in the fingers (paresthesia), tetany or painful tonic muscle spasms, abdominal cramps, muscle cramps, or spasmodic contractions.

BE SAFE! Tetany and laryngospasm are life-threatening symptoms of severe calcium deficiency and must be managed immediately.

Diagnostic Tests

Test	What It Tells	Patient Problems/ Nursing Care
Serum calcium: total calcium including free ionized calcium and calcium bound with protein or organic ions	Increased in hypercalcemia and decreased in hypocalcemia	Knowledge deficit: explain procedures. Patient will need venipuncture.
Serum ionized calcium: unbound calcium; level unaffected by albumin level	Increased in hypercalcemia and decreased in hypocalcemia	Knowledge deficit: explain procedures. Patient will need venipuncture.

Treatment and Nursing Care

Potential Nursing Diagnoses*

Risk for injury
Risk for ineffective airway clearance
Nausea

BE SMART! Monitor calcium levels and provide supplements as prescribed for low calcium levels.

- The goals of hypercalcemia treatment are to reduce the serum calcium level and to identify and correct the underlying cause.
- Furosemide lowers serum calcium as natriuresis occurs.
- Pamidronate reduces calcium levels by decreasing phosphate release from bone and increasing calcium excretion by kidneys.
- Nursing care for hypercalcemia focuses on fluid balance and intake.
- If the patient with hypocalcemia has an airway obstruction, endotracheal intubation and mechanical ventilation may be needed to manage laryngospasm.
- Calcium supplements correct the calcium deficiency.
- Magnesium sulfate corrects magnesium deficiency, which must be corrected in order to correct calcium deficiency.
- Nursing care for hypocalcemia centers on instituting proper safety measures, teaching the patient to prevent future episodes, and maximizing patient comfort.

Chloride Imbalance—Hyperchloremia and Hypochloremia

Chloride performs a number of essential physiological functions. One is to join with hydrogen to form hydrochloric acid (HCl), which aids in digestion and activates enzymes, such as salivary amylase. Chloride also plays a role in maintaining the serum osmolarity and the body's water balance. Serum chloride excess, *hyperchloremia*, occurs when the serum chloride level is greater than 112 mEq/L. Normal serum chloride level is 101 to 112 mEq/L. Chloride is the major anion in extracellular fluid (ECF). Chloride is regulated in the body primarily through its relationship with sodium. Serum levels of both sodium and chloride often parallel each other. Hyperchloremia, like hypernatremia, causes an increase in the serum osmolarity (the proportion of sodium and chloride ions to water in the ECF). Chloride influences the acid-base balance as well. To maintain acid-base balance, the kidneys excrete chloride or bicarbonate. Each sodium ion that is reabsorbed in the renal tubules reabsorbs either a chloride or a bicarbonate ion, depending on the acid-base balance of the ECF. In metabolic acidosis, the kidney excretes chloride in exchange for bicarbonate. The most common cause of hyperchloremia is body fluid loss, or dehydration, which leads to renal retention of water.

Hypochloremia is a serum chloride level below 95 mEq/L. Chloride deficit leads to a number of physiological alterations such as ECF volume contraction, potassium depletion, intracellular acidosis, and increased bicarbonate generation. Hypochloremia, similar to hyponatremia, also causes a decrease in the serum osmolarity, resulting in a decrease in sodium and chloride ions in proportion to water in the ECF. When there is a body water excess, chloride also may be decreased along with sodium, preventing reabsorption of body water by the kidneys. The most common cause of hypochloremia is gastrointestinal (GI) abnormalities, including prolonged vomiting, nasogastric suctioning, loss of potassium, and diarrhea.

Where It Occurs

- Infants, young children, and elderly people of both sexes are at particular risk for hyperchloremia because they are prone to dehydration.
- Infants, children, and adults of both sexes are at risk for developing hypochloremia, but elderly patients are particularly at risk when they are placed on multiple medications or if they have persistent bouts of vomiting and diarrhea.

Signal Symptoms

- Symptoms of hyperchloremia depend on the source of the chloride imbalance.
- Because most patients who have hyperchloremia also have hypernatremia, signs and symptoms associated with this imbalance may be present, including restlessness, agitation, irritability, muscle twitching, hyperreflexia, and seizures.
- Symptoms of hypochloremia depend on the cause of the chloride deficit; tetany-like symptoms, such as tremors and twitching, may be present, and these neuromuscular symptoms are associated with hyponatremia.

BE SAFE! Be particularly vigilant for signs of neurological dysfunction.

Diagnostic Tests

Test	What It Tells	Patient Problems/ Nursing Care
Serum chloride	Elevated levels indicate hyperchloremia, and decreased levels indicate hypochloremia	Knowledge deficit: explain procedures. Patient will need venipuncture.
Serum osmolarity	Elevated levels indicate hyperchloremia, and decreased levels indicate hypochloremia	Knowledge deficit: explain procedures. Patient will need venipuncture.

Treatment and Nursing Care

Potential Nursing Diagnoses*

Fluid volume deficit
Altered protection
Disturbed thought processes
Risk for injury

BE SMART! Careful monitoring of fluid and electrolyte status is critical.

- Sodium bicarbonate is used for hyperchloremia because it corrects metabolic acidosis.
- Nursing strategies include maintaining both safety measures for patients who develop neuromuscular weakness or lethargy and adequate airway, breathing, and circulation.
- Treatment of hypochloremia involves treating the underlying cause and replacing the chloride.
- Potassium chloride (KCl) and ammonium chloride replace needed electrolytes, particularly in metabolic alkalosis.
- Nursing strategies include maintaining both safety measures for patients who develop neuromuscular symptoms and adequate airway, breathing, and circulation.

Diabetes Insipidus

The disorder diabetes insipidus (DI) is characterized by excretion of large amounts of dilute urine. Neoplasms, infiltrative lesions, malformations, and neurosurgical procedures in the area of the pituitary gland are the most common causes of DI. DI can be of central (neurogenic) or renal (nephrogenic) origin. In central DI, excess urine is caused by insufficient amounts of antidiuretic hormone (ADH, also known as plasma vasopressin). Renal DI occurs when the kidney has a decreased responsiveness to ADH.

Normally, body water balance is partially regulated by ADH, which is produced in the hypothalamus and is released from the posterior pituitary gland when body fluids become more concentrated than usual (serum osmolarity >283 mOsm/L). ADH causes water reabsorption in the distal portions of the nephron of the kidney by increasing the number of pores in the distal tubular system to allow for water reabsorption. ADH deficiency leads to little or no reabsorption; as a consequence, dilute urine formed in more proximal parts of the nephron is excreted essentially unchanged. The loss of solute-free water causes mild dehydration, a rise in plasma osmolality, and the stimulation of thirst.

Where It Occurs

- Males are slightly more likely than females to develop DI.
- Children and elderly people are more likely to experience complications from DI.

Signal Symptoms

- Polyuria, polydipsia, and nocturia.
- Signs of dehydration: poor skin turgor, thirst, hypotension.
- In infants, the most common signs are crying and irritability, hyperthermia, and weight loss.

BE SAFE! As long as water is available and the patient is awake enough to drink, serious complications are unusual.

Diagnostic Tests

Test	What It Tells	Patient Problems/ Nursing Care
Urine osmolality	Decreased osmolality indicates excretion of dilute urine in spite of dehydration and hypernatremia due to underproduction of ADH	Knowledge deficit: explain procedures.
Blood osmolality	Increased osmolality indicates water loss in the urine and hemoconcentration	Knowledge deficit: explain procedures. Patient will need venipuncture.

Treatment and Nursing Care

Potential Nursing Diagnoses*

Fluid volume deficit
Imbalanced nutrition, less than body requirements
Impaired urinary elimination

BE SMART! Teach patient to take extra care in hot weather, which might lead to dehydration and increased symptoms.

- The most important aspect of DI treatment is to treat the underlying cause.
- Aqueous vasopressin is a supplement that provides hormone in ADH deficiency.
- Chlorpropamide (Diabinese) reduces urine output by 30% to 70%.
- The most important nursing interventions focus on maintaining an adequate balance of fluid intake and output.

Magnesium Imbalance—Hypermagnesemia and Hypomagnesemia

Hypermagnesemia occurs when the serum magnesium concentration is greater than 2.7 mg/dL (2.3 mEq/L), but signs and symptoms do not occur until the magnesium reaches 4 mg/dL. The normal serum magnesium level is 1.7 to 2.7 mg/dL (1.4–2.3 mEq/L). Magnesium is found in the bones: 1% is located in the extracellular compartment, and the remainder is found within the cells. Magnesium plays an important role in neuromuscular function. It also has a role in several enzyme systems, particularly the metabolism of carbohydrates and proteins, as well as maintenance of normal ionic balance (it triggers the sodium-potassium pump), osmotic pressure, myocardial functioning, and bone metabolism. Because the kidneys can excrete large amounts of magnesium (>5,000 mg/day), either the patient has to ingest extraordinary amounts of magnesium or the glomerular filtration of the kidneys needs to be very depressed for the patient to develop hypermagnesemia.

Hypomagnesemia occurs when the serum magnesium concentration is less than 1.7 mg/dL (1.4 mEq/L). Deficits of magnesium lead to deficits in calcium, and the two electrolyte imbalances are difficult to differentiate. The hypocalcemia that accompanies hypomagnesemia cannot be corrected unless the magnesium is replaced. Hypomagnesemia is also a stimulus for renin release, which leads to aldosterone production, potassium wasting, and hypokalemia. Because magnesium regulates calcium entry into cells, consequences of magnesium deficiency include ventricular dysrhythmias, an enhanced digitalis toxicity, and sudden cardiac death. Deficits in potassium and calcium potentiate the dysrhythmogenic effect of low magnesium. The primary sources of magnesium deficit are reduced intestinal absorption and increased renal excretion.

Where It Occurs

■ Hypermagnesemia may occur at any age, in both sexes, and in all races and ethnicities, but it is seen much more frequently in the older patient with chronic renal failure.

■ Anyone with a chronic illness that causes malabsorption or renal loss of magnesium is susceptible to hypomagnesemia, but pregnant women with toxemia are particularly at risk, as are the elderly who are placed on diuretic therapy and people with cancer who are taking chemotherapy.

Signal Symptoms

- Hypermagnesemia: muscle weakness and fatigue; palpitations or dizziness, depression, lethargy, thirst, muscle weakness, or even paralysis may also occur.
- Hypomagnesemia: Muscular changes, such as tetany, spasticity, or tremors; seizures, mood changes, irritability, confusion, hallucinations, psychosis, and depression.

BE SAFE! Make sure that the patient has an open airway and adequate breathing.

Diagnostic Tests

Test	What It Tells	Patient Problems/ Nursing Care
Serum magnesium	Excess of magnesium ions indicates hypermagnesemia; deficit of magnesium ions indicates hypomagnesemia	Knowledge deficit: explain procedures. Patient will need venipuncture.
Electrocardiogram	Magnesium excess leads to alterations in generation and conduction of the action potential	Knowledge deficit: explain procedures. Patient will need venipuncture.
Serum calcium: total calcium, including free ionized calcium and bound calcium	Deficit of calcium below normal levels in the extracellular fluid compartment indicates hypomagnesemia	Knowledge deficit: explain procedures. Patient will need venipuncture.

Treatment and Nursing Care

Potential Nursing Diagnoses*

Risk for injury
Ineffective airway clearance
Imbalanced nutrition
Activity intolerance

- To treat hypermagnesemia, all medications containing magnesium are discontinued.
- Furosemide (Lasix) promotes excretion of magnesium and water by interfering with chloride-binding transport system and inhibiting sodium and chloride reabsorption in the kidneys.
- Calcium gluconate 10% antagonizes the effects of magnesium and counteracts neuromuscular effect.
- Nursing care for hypermagnesemia focuses on maintaining the patient's airway, breathing, and circulation until the magnesium levels return to normal.
- In severe hypomagnesemia, the patient needs IV or intramuscular magnesium replacement with magnesium sulfate (MgSO4).
- Magnesium gluconate (Almora) is given when the patient is mildly depleted (magnesium >1 mEq/L and patient is asymptomatic).
- The patient's safety is the primary nursing concern.

Metabolic Acidosis

The hydrogen ion concentration ($[H^+]$) of the body, described as the pH or negative log of the $[H^+]$ is maintained in a narrow range to promote health and homeostasis. The body has many regulatory mechanisms that counteract even a slight deviation from normal pH. Acid-base imbalance can alter many physiological processes and lead to serious problems and, if left untreated, to coma and death. A pH below 7.35 is considered acidosis.

Metabolic acidosis results from any nonpulmonary condition that leads to an excess of acids over bases. Renal patients with chronic acidemia may show signs of skeletal problems as calcium and phosphate are released from bone to help with the buffering of acids. Children with chronic acidosis may show signs of impaired growth. Chronic renal disease results in decreased acid excretion and is the most common cause of chronic metabolic acidosis. Other causes include ketoacidosis, lactic acidosis, and ingestion of acids.

Where It Occurs

- Metabolic acidosis from severe diarrhea can occur at any age, but children and the elderly are at greater risk because of associated fluid imbalances.
- Young women are at an increased risk of metabolic acidosis because of the popular fad diets of starvation.
- Patients with type 1 diabetes mellitus are at risk for ketoacidosis.

Signal Symptoms

- Seizure activity, starvation, shock, acid ingestion, diarrhea, nausea, vomiting, anorexia, abdominal pain, and dehydration are all associated with metabolic acidosis.
- Dyspnea with activity or at rest, as well as weakness, fatigue, headache, or confusion may also occur.
- Nocturia, polyuria, pruritus, and anorexia.

BE SAFE! If patient's mental status is deteriorating, make sure s/he has an open airway and adequate breathing.

Diagnostic Tests

Test	What It Tells	Patient Problems/ Nursing Care
Arterial blood gases	Decreased pH level indicates metabolic acidosis	Knowledge deficit: explain procedures. Patient will need arterial puncture: warn patient that the procedure is painful.

Treatment and Nursing Care

Potential Nursing Diagnoses*

Ineffective health maintenance
Ineffective airway clearance
Fatigue
Risk for trauma

- The highest priority for all patients with acid-base imbalances is to maintain the adequacy of airway, breathing, and circulation.
- Sodium bicarbonate may be administered to treat normal anion gap metabolic acidosis but is controversial in treating increased anion gap metabolic acidosis.
- Assess for teaching needs depending on the underlying cause of acidosis.

Metabolic Alkalosis

The hydrogen ion concentration ($[H^+]$) of the body, described as the pH or negative log of the $[H^+]$, is maintained in a narrow range to promote health and homeostasis. The body has many regulatory mechanisms that counteract even a slight deviation from normal pH. Acid-base imbalance can alter many physiological processes and lead to serious problems and, if left untreated, to coma and death. A pH above 7.45 is alkalosis.

Metabolic alkalosis results from one of two mechanisms: an excess of bases or a loss of acids. Patients with a history of congestive heart failure and hypertension, who are on sodium-restricted diets and diuretics, are at greatest risk for metabolic alkalosis. Metabolic alkalosis can also be caused by prolonged vomiting, gastrointestinal surgery, hyperaldosteronism, and diuretic therapy.

Where It Occurs

- Metabolic alkalosis is a common disorder of adult hospitalized patients.
- Elderly patients are at risk for metabolic alkalosis because of their delicate fluid and electrolyte status.
- Young women who practice self-induced vomiting to lose weight are also at risk for developing metabolic alkalosis.
- Middle-aged men and women with chronic hypercapnia respiratory failure are at risk for metabolic alkalosis if their $Paco_2$ levels are rapidly decreased with mechanical ventilation, corticosteroids, or antacids.

Signal Symptoms

- Possible symptoms include lightheadedness, agitation, muscle weakness, cramping, twitching or tingling, circumoral paresthesia, anorexia, nausea, vomiting.
- Symptoms of hypokalemia: weakness, myalgia, polyuria, and cardiac arrhythmias. Symptoms of hypocalcemia: irritability, tingling, muscle spasms.
- Hypoventilation.

> **BE SAFE!** Hypoventilation may lead to impaired breathing and respiratory arrest.

Diagnostic Tests

Test	What It Tells	Patient Problems/ Nursing Care
Arterial blood gases	Increased pH indicates metabolic alkalosis	Knowledge deficit: explain procedures. Patient will need arterial puncture: warn patient that the procedure is painful.

Treatment and Nursing Care

Potential Nursing Diagnoses*

Ineffective health maintenance
Ineffective airway clearance
Fatigue
Nausea

> **BE SMART!** Monitor electrolytes, particularly calcium and potassium levels, and assess for symptoms of hypokalemia and hypercalcemia.

- The highest priority for all patients with acid-base imbalances is to maintain the adequacy of airway, breathing, and circulation.
- Pharmacologic therapy may include IV saline solutions, potassium supplements, histamine antagonists, and carbonic anhydrase inhibitors.

- Histamine H_2 receptor antagonists, particularly cimetidine and ranitidine, reduce the production of hydrochloric acid in the stomach and may prevent the occurrence of metabolic alkalosis in patients with nasogastric suctioning and vomiting.
- Assess patient for educational needs depending on the underlying cause.

Phosphate Imbalance—Hyperphosphatemia and Hypophosphatemia

Phosphorus is one of the primary intracellular ions in the body. It is found as both organic phosphorus and inorganic phosphorus salts. Phosphate plays a critical role in all of the body's tissues. It is an important structural element in the bones and is essential to the function of muscle, red blood cells, and the nervous system. It is responsible for bone growth and interacts with hemoglobin in the red blood cells, promoting oxygen release to the body's tissues. Phosphate is responsible for promotion of white blood cell phagocytic action and is important in platelet structure and function. It also acts as a buffering agent for urine. In one of its most important roles, phosphate is critical for the production of adenosine triphosphate, the chief energy source of the body. Approximately 85% of body phosphorus is in bone, and most of the remainder is intracellular; only 1% is in the extracellular fluid. Phosphorus is absorbed primarily in the jejunum from foods such as red meats, fish, poultry, eggs, and milk products. Phosphate is regulated by the kidneys; 90% of phosphate excretion occurs by the renal route and 10% by the fecal route. Phosphate is also regulated by vitamin D and by parathyroid hormone. Phosphorus levels are inversely related to calcium levels.

Normal serum phosphate levels are 2.5 to 4.5 mg/dL, whereas intracellular phosphorus levels are as high as 300 mg/dL. Hyperphosphatemia occurs when serum phosphorus levels exceed 4.5 mg/dL. The primary cause of hyperphosphatemia is decreased phosphorus excretion because of renal insufficiency or renal failure (acute or chronic).

Hypophosphatemia occurs when the serum phosphorus levels fall below 1.7 mEq/L (2.5 mg/dL). Patients with moderate hypophosphatemia (1.0–2.5 mg/dL) are usually asymptomatic and require no treatment except to manage the underlying cause; patients with severe hypophosphatemia (<1 mg/dL) need more aggressive treatment to prevent complications. The many causes of hypophosphatemia include dietary changes, gastrointestinal abnormalities, drug interactions, hormonal changes, and cellular changes.

Where It Occurs

- While hyperphosphatemia has no racial or ethnic predilection, African Americans, people of Hispanic origin, and Native Americans have a disproportionately high prevalence of renal failure, which can result in hyperphosphatemia.
- Hypophosphatemia can occur at any age, across both sexes, and in all races and ethnicities. People with chronic alcohol abuse usually have low levels of phosphorus.

Signal Symptoms

- Hyperphosphatemia (similar to hypocalcemia): muscle cramps, tingling, tetany; often have symptoms related to renal failure such as fatigue, nausea, vomiting, anorexia, sleep disturbance.
- Patients with hyperphosphatemia may develop tetanus.
- Hypophosphatemia: tremors, hyporeflexia, paresthesia, weak and irregular pulse, weight loss, and fatigue.

BE SAFE! The greatest risk with tetany associated with hyperphosphatemia is laryngospasm and airway compromise.

Diagnostic Tests

Test	What It Tells	Patient Problems/ Nursing Care
Serum phosphorus	Elevated levels indicate hyperphosphatemia, and decreased levels indicate hypophosphatemia	Knowledge deficit: explain procedures. Patient will need venipuncture.
Serum calcium	Decreased levels indicate hyperphosphatemia	Knowledge deficit: explain procedures. Patient will need venipuncture.
Urine phosphorus	Decreased levels indicate hypophosphatemia	Knowledge deficit: explain procedures.

Potential Nursing Diagnoses*

Imbalanced nutrition, more or less than body requirements
Ineffective airway clearance
Fatigue
Anxiety

> **BE SMART!** Medication and fluid management are critical for
> electrolyte imbalance.

- Medical treatment of hyperphosphatemia is aimed at managing the underlying disease process.
- Acetazolamide (Diamox) increases renal excretion of phosphorus.
- Phosphate-binding agents cause phosphate binding in the gastrointestinal tract, thereby decreasing serum phosphate levels.
- Nursing care for hyperphosphatemia focuses on educating the patient and identifying any developing symptoms of the disorder in at-risk patients.
- The most important treatment goals for hypophosphatemia are to replace the phosphorus and to correct the underlying cause of the phosphorus deficit.
- Phosphate supplements are used to replace phosphorus.
- Nursing care for both hyperphosphatemia and hypophosphatemia focuses on maintaining an open airway, adequate breathing, and a safe environment.

Respiratory Acidosis

The hydrogen ion concentration ($[H^+]$) of the body, described as the pH or negative log of the $[H^+]$, is maintained in a narrow range to promote health and homeostasis. The body has many regulatory mechanisms that counteract even a slight deviation from normal pH. Acid-base imbalance can alter many physiological processes and lead to serious problems and, if left untreated, to coma and death. A pH below 7.35 is considered acidosis.

Respiratory acidosis is a pH imbalance that results from alveolar hypoventilation and an accumulation of carbon dioxide. It can be classified as either acute or chronic. Acute respiratory acidosis is associated with a sudden failure in ventilation. Chronic respiratory acidosis is seen in patients with chronic pulmonary disease in whom long-term hypoventilation results in a chronic elevation (>45 mm Hg) of $Paco_2$ levels (hypercapnia), which renders the primary mechanism of inspiration, an elevated $Paco_2$, unreliable. The major drive for respiration in chronic pulmonary disease patients becomes a low oxygen level (hypoxemia).

Where It Occurs

■ Patients of all ages are at risk for acute respiratory acidosis when an injury or illness results in alveolar hypoventilation.

Signal Symptoms

■ Early: changes in a patient's behavior, such as signs of confusion, impaired judgment, lack of motor coordination, and restlessness.
■ Late: increased heart rate, headache, lethargy, blurred vision, confusion, nausea.

BE SAFE! Make sure that the patient has an open airway and adequate breathing to reduce the consequences of hypoventilation.

Diagnostic Tests

Test	What It Tells	Patient Problems/ Nursing Care
Arterial blood gases	Decreased pH and increased $Paco_2$ levels indicate respiratory acidosis	Knowledge deficit: explain procedures. Patient will need arterial puncture: warn patient that the procedure is painful.

Treatment and Nursing Care

Potential Nursing Diagnoses*

Impaired gas exchange
Ineffective breathing pattern
Risk for injury
Confusion, acute

BE SMART! Patient will probably need to have oxygen through an
oxygen-delivery system and may need endotracheal intubation and
mechanical ventilation. Be prepared to assist with these procedures.

- The highest priority for all patients with acid-base imbalances is to
  maintain the adequacy of airway, breathing, and circulation.
- Although oxygen therapy is required to treat the hypoxemia that
  accompanies respiratory acidosis, a fraction of inspired air (Fio_2) of
  less than 0.40 is desirable.
- Pharmacologic therapy for respiratory acidosis depends on the cause
  and severity of acidosis.
- The administration of sodium bicarbonate is controversial for a
  pH greater than 7.0. If the pH is below 7.0, sodium bicarbonate
  administration is recommended.
- Complete serial assessments until patient has stabilized.

Respiratory Alkalosis

The hydrogen ion concentration ($[H^+]$) of the body, described as the pH
or negative log of the $[H^+]$, is maintained in a narrow range to promote
health and homeostasis. The body has many regulatory mechanisms that
counteract even a slight deviation from normal pH. Acid-base imbalance
can alter many physiological processes and lead to serious problems and,
if left untreated, to coma and death. A pH above 7.45 is alkalosis.

Respiratory alkalosis is a pH imbalance that results from the excessive loss of carbon dioxide through hyperventilation ($Paco_2$ <35 mm Hg).
Improper use of mechanical ventilators can cause iatrogenic respiratory
alkalosis, whereas secondary respiratory alkalosis may develop from
hyperventilation stimulated by metabolic or respiratory acidosis. Patients

with respiratory alkalosis are at risk for hypokalemia, hypocalcemia, and hypophosphatemia.

Where It Occurs

- The elderly are at an increased risk for respiratory alkalosis because of the high incidence of pulmonary disorders, specifically pneumonia, in the elderly population.
- Older children and adults are at risk for respiratory alkalosis with large-dose salicylate ingestion (metabolic acidosis leads to respiratory compensation).

Signal Symptoms

- Hyperventilation, tachypnea.
- Lightheadedness, anxiety, inability to concentrate, or confusion, due to decreased $Paco_2$ levels (hypocapnia), which may lead to decreased cerebral perfusion.
- Muscle cramps, spasms, tingling (paresthesia) of the extremities, circumoral numbness, nausea, and vomiting

BE SAFE! Patients who are anxious tend to have even more rapid respirations. Create a calming environment and try to help patient relax.

Diagnostic Tests

Test	What It Tells	Patient Problems/ Nursing Care
Arterial blood gases	Increased pH and decreased $Paco_2$ levels indicate respiratory alkalosis	Knowledge deficit: explain procedures. Patient will need arterial puncture: warn patient that procedure is painful.

Treatment and Nursing Care

Potential Nursing Diagnoses*

Impaired gas exchange
Ineffective breathing pattern

Risk for injury
Confusion, acute
Anxiety

BE SMART! Check calcium levels and make sure calcium is adequate. Hyperventilation can magnify calcium imbalance.

- The highest priority for all patients with acid-base imbalances is to maintain the adequacy of airway, breathing, and circulation.
- Because the most common cause of respiratory alkalosis is anxiety, reassurance and sedation may be all that are needed.
- Pharmacologic therapy most likely includes the administration of anti-anxiety medications and potassium supplements.
- If the cause of the hyperventilation is hypoxemia, oxygen therapy is needed.

Sodium Imbalance—Hypernatremia and Hyponatremia

Sodium is the most abundant cation in the body, and about 30% of the total body sodium, called *silent sodium*, is bound with bone and other tissues; the remaining 70%, called *exchangeable sodium*, is dissolved in the extracellular fluid (ECF) compartment or in the compartments in communication with the ECF compartment. Sodium has five essential functions: it maintains the osmolarity of the ECF; it maintains ECF volume and water distribution; it affects the concentration, excretion, and absorption of other electrolytes, particularly potassium and chloride; it combines with other ions to maintain acid-base balance; and it is essential for impulse transmission of nerve and muscle fibers.

Hypernatremia is a condition in which the serum sodium concentration is greater than 145 mEq/L (normal range is 136–145 mEq/L). It usually occurs when there is an excess of sodium in relation to water in the ECF compartment, resulting in hyperosmolarity of the ECF, which produces a shift in water from the cells to the ECF. The result is cellular dehydration. Three different manifestations of hypernatremia have been described on the basis of the ratio of total body water (TBW) to total body sodium: hypovolemic hypernatremia, hypervolemic hypernatremia, and euvolemic hypernatremia.

Hyponatremia is a serum sodium concentration less than 135 mEq/L. Hyponatremia is the most common of all electrolyte disorders. As serum sodium decreases, water in the ECF moves into the cells. There is less sodium available to move across an excitable membrane, which results in delayed membrane depolarization. Central nervous system cells are most likely to be affected by these changes. Four different manifestations of hyponatremia have been described on the basis of the ratio of TBW to total body sodium: hypovolemic hyponatremia, hypervolemic hyponatremia, euvolemic hyponatremia, and redistributive hyponatremia.

Where It Occurs

- Hypernatremia is most likely to occur in infants, elderly people (especially those institutionalized), persons with mental or physical impairment, or debilitated patients. They may report reduced fluid intake or increase in salt intake.
- Hyponatremia can occur in any age group, in all races and ethnicities, and in both sexes; however, it is more common in infants, young children, elderly people, and debilitated patients because these groups are more likely to experience variation in the TBW.

Signal Symptoms

- Hypernatremia: polyuria moving to oliguria, thirst, dry mouth, poor skin turgor, orthostatic blood pressure changes, weight loss, weakness, lethargy, irritability, confusion, abnormal speech, seizures, nystagmus, jerking movements.
- Hyponatremia: nausea, vomiting, diarrhea, abdominal cramps, headache, dizziness, weight loss, anorexia and changes in mental status or behavior such as confusion, a flat affect, and personality changes.

BE SAFE! Low or high sodium is a significant neurological problem that needs to be corrected promptly but carefully with fluid and electrolyte supplementation.

Diagnostic Tests

Test	What It Tells	Patient Problems/ Nursing Care
Serum sodium	Elevated levels indicate hypernatremia; decreased levels indicate hyponatremia	Knowledge deficit: explain procedures. Patient will need venipuncture.
Blood urea nitrogen (BUN)	Conditions that lead to dehydration and fluid loss, such as hypernatremia, may elevate BUN because of decreased renal blood flow and abnormal absorption of urea back into the blood	Knowledge deficit: explain procedures. Patient will need venipuncture.
Serum osmolarity	Hyponatremia leads to hemodilution, showing a decrease in the ratio of water to particles	Knowledge deficit: explain procedures. Patient will need venipuncture.

Treatment and Nursing Care

Potential Nursing Diagnoses*

Deficient or excess fluid volume
Disturbed thought processes
Acute confusion
Pain (acute)
Risk for injury

BE SMART! Make sure that you have a patent intravenous system to deliver fluid and electrolytes.

- The treatment goal for hypernatremia is to decrease the total body sodium and replace the fluid loss.
- If the patient cannot tolerate fluids, an IV hypotonic electrolyte solution (0.2% or 0.45% sodium chloride) or salt-free solution is usually ordered.

- Nursing care for hypernatremia includes monitoring fluid balance and observing for changes in mental status.
- The course of treatment for hyponatremia depends on the cause; the goal is to correct the TBW-to-sodium ratio.
- IV hypertonic solutions (3 to 5% sodium chloride) are used to correct the sodium deficit.
- Nursing care for hyponatremia focuses on monitoring fluid balance and maintaining a safe, stable environment.

Syndrome of Inappropriate Antidiuretic Hormone

Syndrome of inappropriate antidiuretic hormone (SIADH), a disorder of the posterior pituitary gland, is a condition of excessive release of antidiuretic hormone (ADH) that results in excessive water retention and hyponatremia. SIADH occurs when ADH secretion is activated by factors other than hyperosmolarity or hypovolemia. Excess ADH secretion increases renal tubular permeability and reabsorption of water into the circulation, resulting in excess extracellular fluid volume, reduced plasma osmolality, increased glomerular filtration rates, and decreased sodium levels. Without treatment, SIADH can lead to life-threatening complications. Water intoxication accompanied by sodium deficit may lead to free water movement into cerebral cells, which can cause cerebral edema and result in coma and even death.

Where It Occurs

- Both children and adults are at risk.
- There are no known racial or ethnic considerations.
- Females seem more at risk than males for hyponatremia.

Signal Symptoms

- Hyponatremia: fatigue, weakness, or headaches progressing to confusion, decreased level of consciousness, seizures, coma; nausea, vomiting, muscle weakness.

- Life-threatening symptoms such as seizures may indicate acute water excess, whereas nausea, muscle twitching, headache, and weight gain are more indicative of chronic water accumulation.

BE SAFE! The most severe, life-threatening signs of SIADH are not fluid overload and pulmonary congestion but rather the central nervous system effects from acute sodium deficiency.

Diagnostic Tests

Test	What It Tells	Patient Problems/ Nursing Care
Urine osmolality	Increased osmolality is the result of the excretion of inappropriately concentrated urine and hyponatremia caused by overproduction of ADH	Knowledge deficit: explain procedures.
Blood osmolality	Water loss in urine and hypernatremia leads to hemoconcentration	Knowledge deficit: explain procedures. Patient will need venipuncture.

Treatment and Nursing Care

Potential Nursing Diagnoses*

Fluid volume excess
Disturbed through process
Fatigue
Imbalanced nutrition
Pain (acute)

BE SMART! Correct sodium carefully to prevent fluid shifts.

- Restoration of normal electrolyte and fluid balance and normal body fluid concentration are the treatment goals. In many patients this can be done with a strict fluid restriction.
- Vasopressin receptor antagonists block vasopressin receptors and are used for hypervolemic and euvolemic (normal volume) hyponatremia when the serum sodium level is less than 125 mEq/L and when

hyponatremia is symptomatic and there has been inadequate response to fluid restriction.

■ Diuretics remove excess fluid volume.

■ If the patient is at risk for airway compromise because of low serum sodium levels or seizure activity, maintaining a patent airway is the primary nursing concern. Strict intake and output, with adherence to fluid restrictions, is essential. Remind patient and family that the fluid restriction is therapeutic and necessary to increase serum sodium.

Acute Alcohol Withdrawal

Alcohol withdrawal is a pattern of physiological responses to the discontinuation of alcohol. Most central nervous system (CNS) depressants produce similar responses, but alcohol is the primary substance in which withdrawal is life threatening, especially if delirium tremens (DTs) occurs and is left untreated.

Withdrawal symptoms should be anticipated with any patient who has been drinking the alcohol equivalent of a six-pack of beer on a daily basis for a period of 6 months; patients with smaller body sizes who have drunk less may exhibit the same symptoms. Alcohol withdrawal involves CNS excitation, respiratory alkalosis, and low serum magnesium levels, leading to an increase in neurological excitement. The primary pathophysiological mechanism is exposure to and then withdrawal of alcohol to neuroreceptors in the brain, which changes receptor interaction with neuroreceptors such as gamma-aminobutyric acid, glutamate, and opiates. Early-stage withdrawal usually occurs within 48 hours of the patient's last drink, with generally mild symptoms. Late-stage alcohol withdrawal, or alcohol withdrawal delirium, usually begins 72 to 96 hours after the patient's last drink but can occur up to 2 weeks later. It occurs in approximately 5% of all patients hospitalized with alcohol dependence and is the most acute phase of alcohol withdrawal.

Where It Occurs

- Approximately 70% of people who are alcohol dependent are males, but women are more likely than men to hide dependency.
- Ethnicity and race have no known effects on alcohol withdrawal.

Signal Symptoms

- Recent agitation, restlessness, anxiety, disorientation, and tremors are signs of the onset of early-stage alcohol withdrawal.
- Humorous comments about alcohol intake are an early sign.
- Increased temperature, blood pressure, and heart rate.

BE SAFE! Treat alcohol withdrawal early. Delirium tremens and seizures can be life threatening.

Diagnostic Tests

Test	What It Tells	Patient Problems/ Nursing Care
Blood alcohol concentration	Positive result indicates alcohol use	Knowledge deficit: explain procedures. Patient will need venipuncture.
Liver function gamma-glutamyl transpeptidase	Elevated levels are evidence of liver disease or alcohol dependence	Knowledge deficit: explain procedures. Patient will need venipuncture.

Treatment and Nursing Care

Potential Nursing Diagnoses*

Risk for fluid volume deficit
Ineffective airway clearance
Nutrition: less than body requirements
Ineffective health maintenance

BE SMART! If they can tolerate fluids by mouth, hydrate patients with fruit juices or water to avoid dehydration.

- Although sedation should prevent withdrawal, if withdrawal occurs, patients often require intravenous hydration with fluid requirements ranging from 4 to 10 L in the first 24 hours.
- Thiamine and multivitamin supplements counter the effects of nutritional deficiencies.
- Benzodiazepine family of medications manages alcohol withdrawal through its sedating effect and its ability to control the tremors or seizures.
- Managing fluid volume deficit is a top priority in nursing care.

Bacteremia and Sepsis

Bacteremia occurs when bacteria infiltrate the blood. Many cases of bacteremia are benign and resolve spontaneously, but some lead to serious infections such as pneumonia, osteomyelitis, cellulitis, and meningitis.

Sepsis is symptomatic bacteremia. *Septic shock* is a clinical syndrome associated with severe systemic infection. It is a sepsis-induced shock with hypotension despite adequate fluid replacement. Patients have perfusion abnormalities, including lactic acidosis, oliguria (urine output <400 mL/day), or an acute alteration in mental status. Often septic shock is characterized by decreased organ perfusion, hypotension, and organ dysfunction.

Where It Occurs

- Children under 3 are at a high risk for developing bacteremia. Elderly are at risk for bacteremia, sepsis, and septic shock. Elderly men may develop urosepsis due to obstruction caused by prostatic hypertrophy.
- At-risk patients include those with diabetes, systemic lupus erythematosus, or alcoholism or patients on corticosteroids.

Signal Symptoms

- Fever is a common symptom of bacteremia. Pain may occur in the abdomen (indicating possible peritonitis, Crohn's disease, appendicitis, cholecystitis, or pancreatitis) or costovertebral angle (CVA) tenderness (indicating possible acute pyelonephritis).
- Common symptoms of sepsis include fever, impaired mental status, and increased breathing rate.

BE SAFE! Start antibiotics as soon as they are prescribed.

Diagnostic Tests

Test	What It Tells	Patient Problems/ Nursing
White blood cell (WBC) count	Increased WBC count is consistent with a diagnosis of bacteremia	Knowledge deficit: explain procedures. Patient will need venipuncture.
Culture and sensitivities	Presence or absence of bacteria	Knowledge deficit: explain procedures. Patient will need venipuncture.

Treatment and Nursing Care

Potential Nursing Diagnoses*

Risk for infection
Hyperthermia
Pain (acute)
Imbalanced nutrition (less than body requirements)
Fluid volume deficit

BE SMART! Remember that the people who are most vulnerable for serious infections are the very old and the very young.

- If culture and sensitivity is positive for bacteria, administer antibiotics as prescribed.
- Ibuprofen and acetaminophen may be used to reduce fever with bacteremia.
- Make sure the patient is adequately hydrated.
- Rest and sleep are important for recovery of infections.

Carbon Monoxide Poisoning

Carbon monoxide (CO) is formed as a by-product of burning organic compounds and is a threat to life because of impaired oxygen delivery and utilization at the cellular level. It has a stronger affinity for hemoglobin than oxygen (it binds to hemoglobin 230–270 times more strongly than oxygen); therefore, even in small concentrations, elevated CO levels can result in clinically important levels of carboxyhemoglobin (HbCO). CO toxicity has its strongest impact on the body organs with the highest requirement for oxygen, such as the brain and heart. Toxicity, therefore, occurs from cellular hypoxia due to lack of oxygen delivery to the tissues.

Sources of CO include fires, stoves, portable heaters, and improperly vented gas water heaters, kerosene space heaters, and charcoal and hibachi grills. Other sources are automobile exhaust, cigarette smoke, propane and gas engines, and inhalation of methylene chloride vapors in cleaning solutions.

Where It Occurs

- Males make up 74% of accidental deaths by carbon monoxide poisoning not related to fire.
- Accidental exposure: riding in the back of enclosed pickup trucks, swimming behind a motor boat, industrial exposure at paper mills, steel foundries, and plants producing coal products.

Signal Symptoms

- Symptoms are often vague and broad. Most common are headache, dizziness, and nausea.
- Possible symptoms include lethargy, dyspnea during exertion, chest pain, palpitations, confusion, and other personality changes.
- Pallor is typical; classic cherry red color is a very late sign.

BE SAFE! Immediately remove the patient from the area of exposure and institute oxygen therapy with a nonrebreather mask with 100% oxygen.

Diagnostic Tests

Test	What It Tells	Patient Problems/ Nursing Care
HbCO analysis	Elevated levels are consistent with CO poisoning	Knowledge deficit: explain procedures. Patient will need venipuncture.
Arterial blood gas	Pao_2 levels remain in the normal range; oxygen saturation must be directly measured and not calculated	Knowledge deficit: explain procedures. Check for bleeding and pulses distal to the puncture.

Treatment and Nursing Care

Potential Nursing Diagnoses*

Impaired gas exchange
Ineffective breathing pattern

Nausea
Knowledge deficit (sources of CO)

BE SMART! Explore possible cases of accidental exposure: stationary vehicles with malfunctioning exhaust systems or inadequately ventilated interior; use of fuel-burning heaters inside a car, camper, or poorly ventilated room.

- Remove the source of CO; immediately institute oxygen therapy at 100%.
- If necessary, intubation may be performed.
- Comatose patients may need transfer to hyperbaric oxygen center.
- Encourage rest and quiet to minimize oxygen consumption.

Disasters

Natural disasters such as earthquakes, tsunami, and tornados and human-made (technological) disasters such as nuclear power plant meltdown, war, terrorism, and explosions occur somewhere in the world daily. Disaster preparation is an essential part of the health-care system. While both the attack on the World Trade Center and weather disasters have drawn attention to the need for disaster planning, complacency and underestimation of the impact of disasters hinders significant planning and resource allocation. When a disaster strikes, the general population expects public service agencies and other branches of the local, state, or federal government to rapidly mobilize to help the injured and the community in general.

Where It Occurs

- Anywhere in the world.
- Developing nations have a higher human cost because of urban crowding and decreased response systems.

Signal Symptoms

- Disruption of food and water supplies.
- Threatened environmental and social infrastructure.

BE SAFE! Preservation of life and health of exposed individuals are of the highest importance in disasters.

Diagnostic Tests

Air quality, water safety, waste disposal, and radiation levels all might need to be assessed depending on the type of disaster.

Treatment and Nursing Care

Potential Nursing Diagnoses*

Risk for infection
Risk for injury
Imbalanced nutrition
Fear
Anxiety

BE SMART! Planning for all contingencies reduces the negative, overall health effects of a disaster.

- Disasters can be classified by the level of response. Level I: local emergency response contains disaster. Level II: regional response that pools aid from surrounding communities. Level III: local and regional assets are overwhelmed, and statewide/federal aid is required.
- Generally disaster planning goes through four steps: (1) mitigation, (2) planning, (3) response, and (4) recovery.
- Debriefing with all personnel involved (first responders, health-care personnel, security, etc.) will improve future disaster efforts.

Shock, Cardiogenic

Cardiogenic shock occurs when cardiac output is insufficient to meet the metabolic demands of the body, resulting in inadequate tissue perfusion. There are four stages of cardiogenic shock: initial, compensatory, progressive, and refractory. During the initial stage, there is diminished cardiac output without any clinical symptoms. In the compensatory stage, the baroreceptors respond to the decreased cardiac output by stimulating the sympathetic nervous system to release catecholamines to improve myocardial contractility and vasoconstriction, leading to increased venous return and arterial blood pressure. Impaired renal perfusion activates the renin-angiotensin system, whose end-product, angiotensin II, causes sodium and water retention as well as vasoconstriction. The progressive stage follows the compensatory stage if there is no intervention or if the intervention fails to reverse the inadequate tissue perfusion. Compensatory mechanisms, aimed at improving cardiac output and tissue perfusion, place an increased demand on an already compromised myocardium. As tissue perfusion remains inadequate, the cells begin anaerobic metabolism, leading to metabolic acidosis and fluid leakage out of the capillaries and into the interstitial spaces. A decrease in circulating volume and an increase in blood viscosity may cause clotting in the capillaries and tissue death.

As the body releases fibrinolytic agents to break down the clots, disseminated intravascular coagulation (DIC) may ensue. Lactic acidosis causes depression of the myocardium and a decrease in the vascular responsiveness to catecholamines, further reducing cardiac output. Blood pools and stagnates in the capillaries, and the continued increase in hydrostatic pressure causes fluid to leak into the interstitium. Severe cerebral ischemia causes depression of the vasomotor center and loss of sympathetic stimulation, resulting in blood pooling in the periphery, a decrease in preload, and further reduction in cardiac output. If there is no effective intervention at this point, the shock will progress to the refractory stage, when the chance of survival is extremely limited.

Where It Occurs

■ Cardiogenic shock can occur at any age but is more common in the middle-aged and older adult.

■ While the overall incidence of cardiogenic shock is higher in men than in women, the percentage of female patients with myocardial infarction (MI) who develop cardiogenic shock is higher than that of male patients with MI.

Signal Symptoms

■ History of symptoms of an acute MI: crushing, viselike chest pain; heaviness that radiates to the arms, neck, or jaw; discomfort lasting more than 20 minutes and unrelieved by nitroglycerin and rest; nausea, vomiting.

- Early: may be no clinical findings unless the cardiac output can be measured.
- Compensatory stage: altered level of consciousness; sinus tachycardia; the presence of an S3 or S4 gallop rhythm; jugular venous distention; hypotension; low urine output; cool extremities; rapid, deep respirations; pulmonary crackles; pulmonary edema; diaphoresis.

BE SAFE! Cardiogenic shock is an emergency; if circulation is not maintained or re-established, the patient will have a cardiac arrest.

Diagnostic Tests

Test	What It Tells	Patient Problems/ Nursing Care
Hemodynamic monitoring	Elevated filling pressures in the heart and low systolic blood pressure occur in the setting of low cardiac output	Knowledge deficit: explain all procedures.

Treatment and Nursing Care

Potential Nursing Diagnoses*

Decreased cardiac output
Ineffective tissue perfusion (peripheral, cerebral, renal, and cardiopulmonary)
Ineffective breathing pattern
Pain (acute)
Anxiety

BE SMART! Patient will need supportive care and possibly mechanical ventilation. Make sure to provide for adequate rest and mechanisms for communication.

- The primary goal in treating cardiogenic shock is improvement in tissue perfusion and oxygenation.
- Although the patient needs an adequate blood pressure, afterload may also need to be decreased, which may be accomplished with

hemodynamic monitoring and the intra-aortic balloon pump (IABP) or ventricular assist device.

■ Dopamine, norepinephrine, and epinephrine support blood pressure and preserve perfusion pressure to vital organs. Dobutamine improves heart contractility without much effect on heart rate.

■ Diuretics reduce venous return. Generally patients need anticoagulation, thrombolytic, or antiplatelet therapy.

■ Limiting myocardial oxygen consumption is a primary nursing concern.

■ Patient will likely need cardiac rehabilitation with teaching about activity, medications, sexuality, and nutrition.

Shock, Hypovolemic/Hemorrhagic

Hypovolemic shock results from a decreased effective circulating volume of water, plasma, or whole blood and is the most common type of shock in adults and children. External, sudden blood loss resulting from penetrating trauma and severe gastrointestinal bleeding are common causes of hemorrhagic shock. A significant loss of greater than 30% of circulating volume results in a decrease in venous return, which in turn diminishes cardiac output and decreases perfusion to vital organs, causing the symptoms associated with shock. When insufficient oxygen is available to the cells, metabolism shifts from aerobic to anaerobic pathways. In this process, lactic acid accumulates in the tissues, and the patient develops metabolic acidosis. In addition, the tissues do not receive adequate glucose, and they cannot accomplish the removal of carbon dioxide. This disruption in normal tissue metabolism results initially in cellular destruction and, if left uncorrected, death.

The American College of Surgeons separates hypovolemic/hemorrhagic shock into four classifications: Stage I occurs when up to 15% of the circulating volume, or approximately 750 mL, of blood is lost. These patients often exhibit few symptoms because compensatory mechanisms support bodily functions. Stage II occurs when 15% to 30% of the circulating volume, or up to 1,500 mL, of blood is lost. These patients have subtle signs of shock, but vital signs usually remain normal. Stage III occurs when 30% to 40% of the circulating volume, or 1,500 to 2,000 mL, of blood is lost. This patient looks acutely ill. The most severe form of hypovolemic/hemorrhagic shock is stage IV. This patient has lost more than 40% of circulating volume, or least 2,000 mL of blood, and is at risk for exsanguination.

Where It Occurs

- Hypovolemic shock can occur at any age and in both sexes, and there are no specific racial and ethnic considerations.
- Hypovolemic shock is the most common type of shock and occurs with traumatic injury. Young adult males are most commonly affected by multiple trauma.

Signal Symptoms

- Diminished cerebral perfusion (early): restlessness, anxiety, agitation, dizziness, irritability, and confusion.
- Diminished renal perfusion: low urine output; concentrated urine.
- Peripheral signs: cold, clammy skin; weak, rapid pulses; delayed capillary refill, signs of dehydration.

BE SAFE! Four areas are considered to be life threatening: (1) chest (auscultate for decreased breath sounds), (2) abdomen (examine for tenderness or distention), (3) thighs (check for deformities and bleeding into soft tissues), and (4) external bleeding.

Diagnostic Tests

No one specific diagnostic test identifies the degree of hypovolemic shock state. Several laboratory indicators do provide valuable information on the status of the patient, however. These include arterial blood gases, hemodynamic parameters (cardiac output and cardiac index, oxygen delivery, oxygen consumption, central venous pressure, pulmonary capillary wedge pressure, and systemic vascular resistance), blood lactate level, hemoglobin, and hematocrit. Radiographic and imaging studies are important depending on the location of interest and might include chest and abdominal x-rays, transesophageal echocardiography, aortography, computed tomography, magnetic resonance imaging, or focused abdominal sonography for trauma. A pregnancy test should be completed for females of childbearing years and, if positive, followed by pelvic sonography.

Treatment and Nursing Care

Potential Nursing Diagnoses*

Fluid volume deficit
Ineffective tissue perfusion (peripheral)
Ineffective airway clearance
Anxiety

BE SMART! Fluid resuscitation is the most important intervention for the patient after airway and breathing are managed.

- The initial care of the patient with hypovolemic shock follows the ABCs of resuscitation.
- Somatostatin (Zecnil) increases reabsorption of water from the kidney tubules.
- The objective of fluid replacement is to provide for adequate cardiac output to perfuse the tissues. This is usually done through large-bore central IV or peripheral catheters and may be done under pressure. Crystalloid, colloid, and blood products may be used depending on the underlying cause.
- After initial stabilization of airway and breathing, the most important nursing intervention is to ensure timely fluid replacement.

Shock, Septic

Septic shock is a clinical syndrome associated with severe systemic infection. It is a sepsis-induced shock with hypotension despite adequate fluid replacement. Patients have perfusion abnormalities, including lactic acidosis, oliguria (urine output <400 mL/day), and possibly an acute alteration in mental status. Often septic shock is characterized by decreased organ perfusion, hypotension, and organ dysfunction.

The syndrome usually begins with the development of a local infectious process. Bacteria from the local infection enter the systemic circulation and release toxins into the bloodstream. Gram-negative bacteria release endotoxins from their cell membrane as they lyse and die, whereas gram-positive bacteria release exotoxins throughout their life span. These toxins trigger the release of cytokines (proteins released by cells to signal other cells) such as tumor necrosis factor and the interleukins. They also activate phagocytic cells such as the macrophages. The complex chemical reactions lead to multiple system effects. As the syndrome progresses, blood flow becomes more sluggish, tissues become hypoxic, and acidosis develops. Ultimately, major organ systems (such as the lungs, kidneys, liver, and blood coagulation) fail, which leads to multiple organ dysfunction syndrome.

Where It Occurs

- Elderly patients, both men and women, are at high risk because of the immunocompromise associated with the aging process.
- More males than females develop septic shock.

Signal Symptoms

- Early (early hyperdynamic, compensated stage): tachycardia, warm and flushed extremities, fever, normal blood pressure (note that some elderly patients never have a fever).
- Progressive: diastolic blood pressure drops, the pulse pressure widens, the peripheral pulses are bounding; confusion, rapid respiratory rate, and peripheral edema.
- Middle (late hyperdynamic, uncompensated stage): widespread organ dysfunction, reduced urine output, respiratory failure, worsening edema.
- Late: blood pressure falls below 90 mm Hg, cold extremities, hypothermia, multiple organ failure.

BE SAFE! Septic shock is an emergency; if circulation is not maintained, the patient will have a cardiac arrest

Diagnostic Tests

Test	What It Tells	Patient Problems/ Nursing Care
Cultures and sensitivities	Identifies infecting organism in blood, urine, sputum, or wounds, although the bacterium is often not ever identified	Knowledge deficit: explain all procedures.

Treatment and Nursing Care

Potential Nursing Diagnoses*

Risk for infection
Decreased cardiac output
Ineffective tissue perfusion (peripheral, cerebral, renal,
   and cardiopulmonary)
Ineffective breathing pattern
Pain (acute)
Anxiety

> **BE SMART!** Patient will need supportive care and possibly
> mechanical ventilation. Make sure to provide for adequate rest
> and mechanisms for communication.

- The primary goals of treatment in septic shock are to maintain
  oxygen delivery to the tissues and to restore the vascular volume,
  blood pressure, and cardiac output.
- Vasopressors maintain an adequate blood pressure.
- Broad-spectrum antibiotics eradicate bacteria.
- Priorities of nursing care for the patient with septic shock include
  maintaining airway, breathing, and circulation; preventing the spread
  of infection; increasing the patient's comfort; preventing injury; and
  supporting the patient and family.

Extended Spectrum ß-Lactamase (ESBL) Infection

Extended spectrum ß-lactamases (ESBL) are enzymes made by specific bacteria such as *Klebsiella*, *Enterobacter*, and *Escherichia coli*. ESBL-secreting bacteria usually survive in the body, particularly in the gastrointestinal tract, without causing infection, but in people who are immunosuppressed (after organ transplantation, on corticosteroids, with HIV/AIDS) may develop ESBL-related infections. Many ESBL-related infections occur in hospitals, day-care centers, and nursing homes as nosocomial infections. ESBL bacteria may also colonize in patients without causing infection and usually gradually disappear over time without treatment.

These bacteria are resistant to penicillins, cephamycins, and carbapenems (ertapenem) because the ESBL deactivates the drugs' antibacterial properties.

Where It Occurs

- Very old and very young are most at risk for ESBL infections.
- Day-care centers for infants and children.
- Hospitals and nursing homes.
- Patients on long-term antibiotic therapy, especially excessive broad-spectrum medication.
- Presence of indwelling catheters (Foley, central venous, feeding tube).

Signal Symptoms

- Fever, chills, malaise.
- Depends on site of infection. Urinary (burning, urgency, hesitancy); pulmonary (flu-like syndrome, cough, nasal discharge); wounds (discharge, decreased healing).

BE SAFE! Frequent hand washing is one of the best preventive measures for ESBL infections.

Diagnostic Tests

Test	What It Tells	Patient Problems/ Nursing Care
Blood, urine, stool, sputum, or wound cultures	Presence of ESBL bacteria	Knowledge deficit: explain procedures; may require venipuncture.

Treatment and Nursing Care

Potential Nursing Diagnoses*

Risk for infection
Fluid volume deficit
Pain (acute)
Impaired skin integrity

BE SMART! Assess patients who have been on broad-spectrum antibiotics for some time for ESBL-resistant infections.

- Promptly initiate antibiotics, such as third-generation cephalosporins (e.g., cefotaxime, ceftriaxone). Infections caused by ESBL-producing *E. coli* or *Klebsiella* bacteria have the best outcomes when treated with imipenem or meropenem.
- Encourage patients to take the entire prescription of antibiotic rather than stopping when symptoms subside.
- Institute procedures in day-care centers to ensure frequent hand washing and cleansing of countertops.

H1N1 Virus Infection

H1N1 influenza, or swine flu, is an extremely contagious febrile respiratory disease found in pigs. It is rare for the disease to spread to humans, but once it does, the virus can be spread similarly to seasonal influenza by the human-to-human route. The disease generally lasts 4 to 6 days.

Where It Occurs

■ Children seem to be at a higher risk than adults of contracting H1N1.

Signal Symptoms

■ Symptoms are similar to symptoms of seasonal influenza, such as fever, cough, sore throat, body or headaches, chills, fatigue, and gastrointestinal symptoms.
■ Children with severe disease may show the following: tachypnea, dyspnea, cyanosis, apnea, dehydration, irritability, decreased mental status.

BE SAFE! Patients with active disease should remain at home for 7 days to limit the spread of disease. To limit transmission in families, patients should wear a face mask when in close proximity to family members.

Diagnostic Tests

Test	What It Tells	Patient Problems/ Nursing Care
Swab for H1N1 virus	Positive for influenza virus	Knowledge deficit: explain all procedures.

Treatment and Nursing Care

Potential Nursing Diagnoses*

Risk for infection
Activity intolerance
Ineffective breathing pattern
Fluid volume deficit

BE SMART! Most patients recover with supportive therapy, bedrest, and fluids.

- Antiviral medications: oseltamivir and zanamivir.
- Treatment goals include rest, fluid monitoring, and minimizing patient discomfort and symptoms.
- Antipyretics are used to control fever.
- Analgesics are used to control pain.
- Nursing care centers on supportive care, rest, and fluids. Frequent hand washing with soap and water is important along with using alcohol-based hand gels.

Methicillin-Resistant *Staphylococcus aureus* (MRSA) Infection

Community-associated methicillin-resistant *Staphylococcus aureus* (CA-MRSA) colonizes on the skin, particularly the perineal skin and skin around the rectum. It is also present in the gastrointestinal (GI) tract and vagina. In addition to community-acquired infections, MRSA is often related to hospital-acquired nosocomial infections.

The organism is carried to skin sites that provide a portal of entry because of breakdown, wounds, scrapes, surgical sites, or indwelling catheters. Often the transmission occurs via the hands of other people such as health-care providers. The infected wound may become abscessed, with a central core of pus surrounded by a fibrin network. From the abscess, the infection may circulate through the blood and result in infection of organs such as the heart, lungs, or bones and joints. Complications include sepsis and septic shock.

Where It Occurs

- More males than females contract MSRA, probably because they are involved in more traumatic events.
- The very young and the very old have the poorest outcomes.
- People with impaired neutrophil function, eczema, IV drug use, and those on immunosuppressives have increased risk.

Signal Symptoms

- Erythema (reddened rash) and fluid-filled blisters of the skin; skin abscesses.
- Fever, chills, malaise, fatigue, anorexia, emesis, diarrhea, myalgias, shortness of breath.
- Bone and joint tenderness, joint redness and warmth.

BE SAFE! If you suspect skin infection from MRSA, encourage patients to contact a health-care provider immediately for appropriate treatment.

Diagnostic Tests

Test	What It Tells	Patient Problems/ Nursing Care
Blood, urine, skin, wound, GI cultures	Determine the presence of bacteria and the appropriate antibiotic sensitivities	Knowledge deficit: explain procedures. Patient will need venipuncture.

Treatment and Nursing Care

Potential Nursing Diagnoses*

Risk for infection
Fatigue
Pain (acute)

BE SMART! Make sure patients understand that they must take all their antibiotics until the prescription is completely gone.

- Hand washing is essential to prevent nosocomial infections and infection transmission. Work with infection-control specialists to make sure the infection is not transmitted to multiple people.
- Surgical drainage of abscesses as needed.
- Vancomycin is often the antibiotic of choice directed against gram-positive organisms and useful in the treatment of septicemia and skin infections.
- Teach the patient about hand washing, administration of antibiotics, and monitoring the skin sites.

Severe Acute Respiratory Syndrome (SARS) Infection

Severe acute respiratory syndrome (SARS) is a severe, potentially life-threatening viral infection that can have fatal complications. Although it initially presents similarly to the flu, it can progress to more serious respiratory conditions such as pneumonia, respiratory failure, and even death. The mortality rate is higher than that of influenza or other respiratory tract infections.

The viral infection is caused by a virus from the *Coronaviridae* family (the SARS-associated coronavirus [SARS-CoV]), which originated in southern China, then spread to Hong Kong and other countries in 2002. Generally, transmission is droplet based or by direct contact, but it may be transmitted by the fecal-oral route as well. Incubation is usually within 10 days.

Where It Occurs

■ All ages, races, ethnicities, and both sexes can be affected by SARS.

Signal Symptoms

■ Fever, shortness of breath, difficulty breathing, and hypoxia.
■ Cough and wheezing.

BE SAFE! Isolate patient from others, and use good hand-washing techniques to prevent spread of infection.

Diagnostic Tests

Test	What It Tells	Patient Problems/ Nursing Care
Antibody test	Presence of antibodies to the SARS virus indicates infection	Knowledge deficit: explain procedures. Patient will need venipuncture.

Treatment and Nursing Care

Potential Nursing Diagnoses*

Impaired gas exchange
Ineffective breathing pattern
Ineffective airway clearance
Risk for infection

BE SMART! Explain to patients that antibiotics generally are not required for viral infections unless there is an accompanying bacterial infection.

- Treatment specific to SARS has not been developed, and so treatment methods should be implemented as though the patient were suffering from pneumonia. Steroids and antiviral agents may be used when appropriate.
- Ventilation and supplemental oxygen may be needed if the patient's airway becomes compromised.
- Conserve the patient's energy by providing rest to minimize oxygen consumption.

Vancomycin-Resistant *Enterococci* (VRE) Infection

Enterococcus bacteria, *E. faecalis* and *E. faecium*, are associated with nosocomial infections, grow in many hospital environments, and are increasingly resistant to antibiotics such as vancomycin. Vancomycin-resistant *Enterococci* (VRE) have both natural and acquired resistance to vancomycin because of a peptide that does not allow for binding. Therefore, the bacteria can continue with cell wall synthesis and proliferation in spite of vancomycin antibiotic administration (they are vancomycin resistant).

Common VRE infections are in the urinary tract, blood (bacteremia), surgical wounds, peritoneum, and pelvis. They are also associated with indwelling catheters. VRE infections are difficult to treat because of limited treatment options except for newer antibiotics such as quinupristin-dalfopristin, daptomycin, linezolid, and tigecycline. Complications include sepsis and septic shock, endocarditis, and damage to the cardiac valves.

Where It Occurs

- Critical-care patients who have received antibiotics for a long period of time.
- Patients receiving organ transplantation.
- Cancer patients.
- Patients with indwelling catheters and receiving total parenteral nutrition.
- VRE infections are common in elderly and debilitated patients of both sexes.

Signal Symptoms

- Urinary: flank or suprapubic tenderness.
- Systemic: fever, new heart murmur, enlarged spleen, petechiae, Janeway lesions, Osler nodes, Roth spots, organ tenderness.
- Catheter insertion site: redness, drainage, swelling, tenderness.

BE SAFE! Hand washing with antimicrobials is one of the best prevention measures available.

Diagnostic Tests

Test	What It Tells	Patient Problems/ Nursing Care
Blood cultures	To determine the nature and antibiotic sensitivities of bacteria	Knowledge deficit: explain all procedures. Patient will need venipuncture.

Treatment and Nursing Care

Potential Nursing Diagnoses*

Risk for infection
Hyperthermia
Pain (acute and chronic)
Fatigue
Activity intolerance

- Antibiotics should match culture and sensitivities and will likely include nitrofurantoin for urinary tract infections and linezolid, daptomycin, or tigecycline.
- Isolate patient according to recommendations published by the Centers for Disease Control and Prevention.
- Surgical drainage of wounds or abscesses may be necessary.
- For enterococcal endocarditis, valve-replacement surgery may be needed to treat heart failure, valvular abscess, or septic emboli.
- Nursing management focuses on rest and recovery, conservation of energy, medication administration, and patient education.

A

Abdominal aortic aneurysm (AAA), 51–52
Acid-base imbalances
  metabolic acidosis, 309–311
  metabolic alkalosis, 311–313
  respiratory acidosis, 315–317
  respiratory alkalosis, 317–319
Acid-fast bacilli sputum, 48
Acquired immunodeficiency syndrome
  (AIDS), 274–276
Acute alcohol withdrawal, 325–326
Acute erosive gastritis, 119
Acute glomerulonephritis (AGN), 150–152
Acute hemorrhagic gastritis, 119
Acute idiopathic demyelinating
  polyneuropathy, 203–205
Acute infective tubulointerstitial
  nephritis, 164
Acute lymphoblastic leukemia (ALL), 283
Acute myelogenous leukemia (AML), 282
Acute renal failure (ACR), 167–170
Acute respiratory distress syndrome
  (ARDS), 18–19
Addison's disease, 231
Adenocarcinomas, 98–99, 144, 146, 233
Adrenal insufficiency, 231–232
Adult-onset polycystic kidney disease
  (ADPKD), 162
Airway, breathing, and circulation
  (ABCs), 2, 3
Alcohol dependence, 125
Alcohol withdrawal, 325–326
Allergies, 20
Alpha-adrenergic drugs, 159, 161
Alpha-fetoprotein, 103
Amputation, 180–182
Amylase, 255
Anaphylaxis, 263–264
Anemia
  aplastic, 264–266
  iron deficiency, 280–281
  sickle cell, 297–299
Aneurysm
  abdominal aortic, 51–52
  cerebral, 195–197, 223
  thoracic aortic, 44–46

Angina, 52–54
Angiotensin-converting enzyme (ACE)
  inhibitors, 66
Ankle arm index (AAI), 181
Anti-acetylcholine receptor (AChR)
  antibody, 212
Anticholinergics, 160
Anticoagulants, 56, 89, 91
Anticonvulsants, 217
Antidiuretic hormone (ADH), 305, 322–324
Antigen testing, 269
Antimuscarinic drugs, 160
Antinuclear antibody, 294
Antithrombin III, 271
Aortic insufficiency, 92
Aortic stenosis, 92
Aphthous stomatitis, 15–17
Aplastic anemia, 264–266
Appendicitis, 94–95
Arrhythmias, cardiac, 57–58
Arterial blood gases (ABGs), 19, 89, 310, 312,
  316, 318, 329
Arterial occlusive disease, 55–56
Arterial pH, 245
Arteriosclerosis, 67
Arthritis
  osteoarthritis, 182–184
  rheumatoid, 293–295
Arthroplasty, 179–180
Aspirin, 54, 56, 69
Asthma, 19–21
Atherosclerosis, 66, 67
Atrophic gastritis, 119

B

Bacteremia, 326–328
Bariatric surgery, 252–253
Barrett's esophagus, 98–99, 121
Bell's palsy, 192–193
Benign prostatic hyperplasia
  (BPH), 142, 170
Benign prostatic hypertrophy, 142–143, 170
Beta-adrenergic blockers, 162
Biliary duct cancer, 100–102
Biopsy, 9

Bladder
  cancer, 144-146
  neurogenic, 158-160
Blood clots, 87-89
Blood pressure, high, 77-79
Blood osmolality, 306, 323
Blood transfusion reaction, 266-267
Blood urea nitrogen (BUN), 79, 149, 169, 320
Body mass index (BMI), 253
Bone cancer, 174-175
Bone infection, 184-186
Bone marrow aspiration, 288
Bone marrow biopsy, 281, 284, 288, 290
Bowel obstruction, 95-96
Braden scale, 7
Brain
  concussion, 195-197
  encephalitis, 199-201
  cancer, 193-195
Breast cancer, 22-23
Bronchodilators, 21
Burns, 1-3

C
Calcium, 255, 257, 301, 308, 314
Calcium channel blockers, 293
Calcium gluconate, 309
Calcium imbalance, 300-302
Cancer
  bladder, 144-146
  bone, 174-175
  brain, 193-195
  breast, 22-23
  colorectal, 97-98
  esophageal, 98-100
  gallbladder, 100-102
  laryngeal, 24-25
  leukemia, 282-285
  liver, 102-103
  multiple myeloma, 287-289
  oral, 9-10
  pancreatic, 233-234
  pancreatic duct, 100-102
  prostate, 146-148
  stomach, 104-105
  thyroid, 235-237
Candidiasis, oral, 10-12
Canker sores, 15-17
Carbon monoxide poisoning, 328-330

Carboxyhemoglobin levels, 2
Cardiac arrhythmias, 57-58
Cardiac catheterization, 59-60, 65, 93
Cardiac stent procedure, 59-62
Cardiac tamponade, 62-64
Cardiac troponin, 83, 85
Cardiogenic shock, 331-334
Cardiomyopathy, 64-66
Cardiovascular disease
  angina, 52-54
  arterial occlusive disease, 55-56
  cardiac arrhythmias, 57-58
  cardiomyopathy, 64-66
  coronary artery disease, 66-69
  cor pulmonale, 69-71
  heart failure, 75-77
  infective endocarditis, 79-81
  myocardial infarction, 81-84
  valvular heart disease, 92-93
Catecholamines, 161
Catheterization, cardiac, 59-60
Cellulitis, 3-4
Cerebral aneurysm, 195-197, 223
Cerebral concussion, 197-199
Cerebrospinal fluid (CSF), 200, 204, 210
Chest tubes, 26-27
Chloride imbalance, 302-304
Cholecystitis, 117-118
Cholelithiasis, 117-118
Chondrosarcoma, 174
Christmas disease, 272
Chronic lymphocytic leukemia (CLL), 282-285
Chronic myelogenous leukemia (CML), 282-285
Chronic obstructive pulmonary disease (COPD), 27-29, 37
Chronic renal failure (CRF), 148-150
Cirrhosis, 125-127
Cluster headache, 205-207
Colitis, 105-107
Colonoscopy, 107, 108, 110, 124, 134
Colorectal cancer, 97-98
Colostomy, 108-109
Community-associated methicillin-resistant
Staphylococcus aureus (CA-MRSA)
infection, 342-343
Compartment syndrome (CS), 176-177
Concussion, 197-199
Congestive heart failure (CHF), 64
Consumptive coagulopathy, 270-272
Continuous venovenous hemodiafiltration
(CVVHD), 169

Cor pulmonale, 69–71
Coronary artery disease
   (CAD), 66–69
Corticosteroids, 75, 211, 266, 287, 292
Cortisol, 232, 237
C-reactive protein, 189
Creatine kinase isoenzyme, 54
Creatinine, 79, 149, 151, 155, 169
Creatinine clearance, 151
Crescentic nephritis, 151
Crohn's disease (CD), 109–111, 133
Cushing's syndrome, 237–239
Cyproheptadine, 239
Cystometry, 159
Cystoscopy, 145
Cytomegalovirus infection (CMV), 267–269

D

D-dimer, 72, 91, 271
Deep vein thrombosis (DVT), 71–73, 90
Defibrination syndrome, 270–272
Delirium tremens (DTs), 325
Desmopressin, 273
Dexamethasone suppression test, 238
Diabetes insipidus (DI), 305–306
Diabetes mellitus (DM)
   type 1, 239–241, 246
   type 2, 242–244, 246
Diabetic ketoacidosis, 244–246
Dialysis
   hemodialysis, 152–154, 169
   peritoneal, 169
Digoxin, 66
Dilated cardiomyopathy, 64–65
Disasters, 330–331
Disease modifying antirheumatic drugs
   (DMARDs), 295
Disseminated intravascular coagulation
   (DIC), 270–272, 332
Diuretics, 170
Diverticular disease, 111–113
Diverticulitis, 111–113
Diverticulosis, 111–113
Dopamine, 170
Duodenal ulcer, 137

E

Electrolytes, 232
Electrophoresis, 288

Embolism
   fat, 73–75
   pulmonary, 87–89
Empyema, 26
Encephalitis, 199–201
Endomyocardial biopsy, 85
End-stage renal disease (ESRD), 148, 152, 153
Enema, 136
Enzyme-linked immunosorbent assay
   (ELISA), 275
Epidural hematoma, 201–203
Epilepsy, 215–217
Epinephrine, 267
Epistaxis, 12–13
Epstein-Barr virus (EBV), 276
Erythrocyte sedimentation rate (ESR),
   183, 189, 292
Esophageal cancer, 98–100
Esophageal manometry, 122
Esophageal varices, 113–115
Esophagitis, 115–116
Esophagogastroduodenoscopy, 120, 138
Exchangeable sodium, 319
Extended spectrum ß-Lactamase (ESBL)
   infection, 339–340
Extracellular fluid (ECF), 319
Eyes, retinal detachment, 14–15

F

Fasting plasma glucose (FPG), 240, 243
Fat embolism, 73–75
Femoral hernia, 131–132
Fiberoptic bronchoscopy, 2
Fibrin degradation products (FDPs), 270
Fine-needle aspiration (FNA) biopsy, 236
First-degree burns, 1
Flu, 31–33, 340–342
Fludrocortisone, 232
Fluorochrome, 48
Folate, 16
Forced expiratory volume in 1 second
   (FEV_1), 21
Forced vital capacity (FVC), 21
Fourth-degree burns, 1
Fractures
   hip, 177–178
   pelvic, 186–188
Fulminant hepatic failure (FHF), 127
Fulminant hepatitis, 129

Functional residual capacity (FRC), 43
Furosemide (Lasix), 302, 309

G
Gallbladder cancer, 100–102
Gallbladder disease, 117–118
Gallstones, 117
Gastric atrophy, 119
Gastric cancer, 104–105
Gastric ulcer, 137
Gastritis, 118–121
Gastroesophageal reflux disease
  (GERD), 115, 121–123
Gastrointestinal hemorrhage, 123–124
Glomerular filtration rate (GFR), 148
Glomerulonephritis, 150–152
Glucocorticoids, 232, 237, 267, 279
Glucose, 241, 246, 249
Glycosylated hemoglobin, 240, 243, 245
Gonadotrophins, 259
Gram stain, 11
Granulomatous colitis, 109–111
Growth hormone, 259
Guillain-Barré syndrome (GBS), 203–205

H
H1N1 virus infection, 340–342
Headache, 205–207
Heart disease. See Cardiovascular disease
Heart failure (HF), 75–77
Helicobacter pylori infection, 104, 119,
  120, 138
Hematest, 98
Hematology, 105
Hemodialysis, 152–154, 169
Hemophilia, 272–274
Hemorrhage, 278
Hemorrhagic shock, 334–336
Hemothorax, 26, 29–31
Hepatic cirrhosis, 125–127
Hepatic failure, 127–129
Hepatitis, 129–131
Hepatitis A, 130, 131
Hepatitis B, 129, 130, 131
Hepatitis C, 125, 130, 131
Hepatitis D, 130
Hepatocellular carcinoma, 102–103
Hernia, 131–133
Herpes zoster (shingles), 4–6
Hip fracture, 177–178

Histamine (H$_2$) receptor antagonists,
  129, 313
HIV disease, 129, 274–276
Hodgkin's disease, 276–278
Homans sign, 90
Human immunodeficiency virus
  (HIV), 129, 274–276
Hydrogen ions, 309, 311, 315, 317
Hydronephrosis, 154–155
Hydroxyurea, 298
Hypercalcemia, 300–302
Hyperchloremia, 302–304
Hyperglycemia, 246–248
Hyperglycemic hyperosmolar nonketotic
  coma (HHNC), 248–250
Hyperkalemia, 153
Hypermagnesemia, 306–309
Hypernatremia, 319–322
Hyperosmolar hyperglycemic state
  (HHS), 248
Hyperosmolar nonketotic syndrome
  (HNKS), 246
Hyperparathyroidism, 256–258
Hyperphosphatemia, 313–315
Hypertension, 77–79
  pulmonary, 41–43, 69
Hyperthyroidism, 260–262
Hypertrophic cardiomyopathy
  (HCM), 64
Hypertrophic obstructive cardiomyopathy, 64
Hyperviscosity, 289
Hypocalcemia, 300–302
Hypochloremia, 302–304
Hypomagnesemia, 306–309
Hyponatremia, 319–322, 322
Hypoparathyroidism, 256–258
Hypophosphatemia, 313–315
Hypothyroidism, 250, 260–262
Hypovolemic shock, 334–336
Hypoxemia, 41

I
Idiopathic hypertrophic subaortic
  stenosis, 64
Idiopathic proctocolitis. See Ulcerative
  colitis
Idiopathic pulmonary fibrosis
  (IPF), 39
Idiopathic thrombocytopenia purpura
  (ITP), 278–280

Ileostomy, 108–109
Impaired glucose tolerance, 246–248
Infections
    bacteremia, 326–328
    cytomegalovirus, 267–269
    extended spectrum ß-Lactamase
        (ESBL), 339–340
    H1N1 virus, 340–342
    Helicobacter pylori, 104, 119, 120, 138
    hepatitis, 129–131
    HIV, 129, 274–276
    infective endocarditis, 79–81
    influenza, 31–33, 340–342
    meningitis, 207–209
    methicillin-resistant *Staphylococcus
        aureus* (MRSA), 342–343
    myocarditis, 84–85
    osteomyelitis, 184–186
    pericarditis, 86–87
    pneumonia, 34–37
    pyelonephritis, 164–165
    severe acute respiratory syndrome
        (SARS), 344–345
    skin, 3–6
    tuberculosis, 47–48
    urinary tract, 172–173
    vancomycin-resistant *Enterococci*
        (VRE), 345–347
    yeast, 10–12
Infective endocarditis (IE), 79–81
Inflammatory bowel disease
    (IBD), 133–134
Influenza, 31–33, 340–342
Inguinal hernia, 131–132
Injuries
    brain, 201–203, 228–230
    burns, 1–3
    cardiac tamponade, 62–64
    spinal cord, 218–219
Insulin, 239, 241, 242, 246
Intermittent hemodialysis (IHD), 169
Intestinal obstruction, 134–136
Intracerebral hemorrhage, 278
Iron, 16
Iron deficiency anemia (IDA), 280–281
Ischemic heart disease, 52–54
Isoniazid, 48

J
Joint replacement, 179–180

K
Kidney stones, 156–157, 165–167
Kidneys
    chronic renal failure, 148–150
    glomerulonephritis, 150–152
    hemodialysis, 152–154
    hydronephrosis, 154–155
    nephrolithiasis, 156–157, 165–167
    polycystic kidney disease, 162–163
    renal failure, 167–170

L
Large-bowel obstructions (LBOs), 95–96
Laryngeal cancer, 24–25
Late-onset hepatic failure, 127
Leukemia, 282–285
Leukocyte esterase, 173
Levothyroxine (Synthroid), 237, 262
Limb amputation, 180–182
Liver
    cancer, 102–103
    cirrhosis, 125–127
    enzymes, 126
    failure, 127–129
    hepatitis, 129–131
Liver function tests, 9, 103, 114, 130
Lower GI bleed (LGIB), 123–124
Lupus erythematosus, 285–287

M
Mafenide acetate, 2
Magnesium gluconate, 309
Magnesium imbalance, 306–309
Magnesium sulfate, 302
Malignant hypertension, 78
Malignant plasmacytoma, 287–289
Mass lesion, 225
Mechanical ventilation, 49–50
Meningitis, 207–209
Mesalamine, 111
Metabolic acidosis, 309–311
Metabolic alkalosis, 311–313
Metered-dose inhalers (MDIs), 21
Methicillin-resistant *Staphylococcus aureus*
    (MRSA) infection, 342–343
Migraine headache, 205–207
Mitotane, 239
Mitral insufficiency, 92
Mitral stenosis, 92

Multiple myeloma, 287–289
Multiple sclerosis (MS), 209–211
Myasthenia gravis (MG), 211–213
Myelomatosis, 287–289
Myocardial infarction (MI), 67, 81–84
Myocarditis, 84–85
Myxedema, 250–251

N
Nasopharyngoscopy, 25
Natural disasters, 330–331
Nephrolithiasis, 156–157, 165–167
Neurogenic bladder, 158–160
Nimodipine, 224
Nitroglycerin, 54
Nosebleed (epistaxis), 12–13

O
Obesity surgery, 252–253
Open pneumothorax, 38
Ophthalmoscopic examination, 15
Oral cancer, 9–10
Oral candidiasis, 10–12
Osteoarthritis (OA), 182–184
Osteomyelitis, 184–186
Osteosarcoma, 174

P
Pamidronate, 302
Pancreatic cancer, 233–234
Pancreatic duct cancer, 100–102
Pancreatitis, 254–256
Panendoscopy, 25
Paragangliomas, 160
Parathyroid hormone (PTH), 256, 258, 300
Parathyroid imbalance, 256–258
Parkinson's disease (PD), 213–215
Partial pressure of oxygen in arterial
    blood, 50, 74
Partial thrombin time, 13, 228
Pelvic fracture, 186–188
Peptic ulcer disease, 137–139
Pericardial sac, 62
Pericarditis, 86–87
Peripheral arterial occlusive disease
    (PAOD), 55–56
Peritoneal dialysis, 169
Peritonitis, 139–141
Petechiae, 74

pH, 309, 311, 315–316, 317
Pheochromocytoma, 160–162
Phosphatase, 175
Phosphate imbalance, 313–315
Phosphorus, 313, 314
Pituitary tumor, 258–260
Plasma cell myeloma, 287–289
Platelet count, 74, 279
Pleural effusion, 26, 33–34
Pneumonia, 34–37
Pneumothorax, 26, 37–39
Polycystic kidney disease, 162–163
Polycythemia, 289–291
Polymerase chain reaction (PCR), 5, 200, 269
Polymyalgia rheumatica (PMR), 188–189
Polyps, 97
Potassium chloride, 304
Pressure ulcer, 6–8
Pressure-cycled ventilators, 49
Primary hypertension, 78
Progressive systemic sclerosis, 291–293
Propylthiouracil (PTU), 262
Prostate
    benign prostatic hypertrophy, 142–143
    cancer, 146–148
    transurethral resection of the, 170–172
Prostate-specific antigen (PSA), 147
Prostatic intraepithelial neoplasia
    (PIN), 146
Proteolytic enzymes, 254
Prothrombin time, 128, 228
Proton pump inhibitors, 120, 123, 138
Pseudoseizures, 215
Pulmonary artery pressure, 42
Pulmonary embolism (PE), 87–89
Pulmonary fibrosis, 39–41
Pulmonary function tests, 50
Pulmonary hypertension, 41–43, 69
Pulmonary vascular resistance (PVR), 42
Pyelonephritis, 164–165

R
Rapidly progressive glomerulonephritis
    (RPGN), 151
Recessive polycystic kidney disease
    (RPKD), 162
Recurrent aphthous ulcers (RAUs), 15–17
Red blood cells (RBCs), 289, 297
Regional enteritis, 109–111, 133
Renal calculi, 156–157, 165–167

Renal failure, 167–170
Respiratory acidosis, 315–317
Respiratory alkalosis, 317–319
Restrictive lung disease, 43–44
Retinal detachment, 14–15
Reverse-transcriptase-polymerase chain reaction, 36
Rheumatoid arthritis (RA), 293–295
Rheumatoid factor, 183
Rifampin, 48
Rocky Mountain spotted fever, 295–296
Rupture, 131–133

S
Sarcomas, 174–175
Scleroderma, 291–293
Secondary hypertension, 78
Second-degree burns, 1
Segmental arterial pressure, 56
Seizure disorder, 215–217
Sepsis, 326–328
Septic shock, 327, 336–338
Serum carcinoembryonic antigen (CEA), 145
Serum cortisol, 232
Serum creatinine, 79, 149, 151, 155, 169
Serum electrolytes, 58, 251
Serum glucose, 247, 249
Serum osmolarity, 247, 251, 304, 320
Severe acute respiratory syndrome (SARS) infection, 344–345
Shingles (herpes zoster), 4–6
Shock
 anaphylactic, 263–264
 cardiogenic, 331–334
 hypovolemic/hemorrhagic, 334–336
 septic, 327, 336–338
Shoulder dislocation, 189–191
Shunting, 88
Sickle cell anemia, 297–299
Sigmoidoscopy, 107, 108, 110
Silent sodium, 319
Silver sulfadiazine, 2
Skin
 burns, 1–3
 infections, 3–6
Small-bowel obstructions (SBOs), 95–96
Smoking cessation, 29
Sodium bicarbonate, 304

Sodium imbalance, 319–322
Somatostatin (Zecnil), 336
Spinal cord injury (SCI), 218–219
Splenectomy, 280
Spontaneous pneumothorax, 38
Squamous cell carcinomas, 9, 98, 144
Status epilepticus, 215
Stenosis, 92–93
Stents, coronary, 60–62
Stomach cancer, 104–105
Stomatitis, 15–17
Stroke, 220–222
Subarachnoid hemorrhage (SAH), 223–224
Subdural hematoma (SDH), 225–226
Subfulminant hepatic failure, 127
Sucralfate (Carafate), 121
Sulfasalazine, 134
Superficial gastritis, 119
Swine flu, 340–342
Syndrome of inappropriate antidiuretic hormone (SIADH), 322–324
Systemic lupus erythematosus (SLE), 150, 285–287

T
Tension pneumothorax, 38
Third-degree burns, 1
Thoracic aortic aneurysm, 44–46
Thromboangiitis obliterans, 55
Thrombophlebitis, 71–73, 90–91
Thromboplastin time, 13
Thyroid
 cancer, 235–237
 disease, 250–251
 hormones, 251, 260
 imbalance, 260–262
Thyroid-stimulating hormone (TSH), 251
Thyrotoxicosis, 260–262
Thyroxine, 251
Time-cycled ventilators, 49
Total lung capacity (TLC), 43
Transient ischemic attacks (TIAs), 220, 227–228
Transurethral resection of the prostate (TURP), 170–172
Traumatic brain injury (TBI), 228–230
Tube thoracostomy, 26–27
Tuberculosis (TB), 47–48

U

Ulcer
  oral, 15–17
  peptic ulcer disease, 137–139
  pressure, 6–8
Ulcerative colitis, 105–107, 133
Umbilical hernia, 131–132
Upper GI bleed (UGIB), 123–124
Urinalysis, 143, 165, 169
Urinary tract infection (UTI), 172–173
Urine culture, 173
Urine osmolality, 306, 323
Uroflowmetry, 143, 159

V

Valvular heart disease, 92–93
Valvular insufficiency, 92
Valvular regurgitation, 92
Valvular stenosis, 92
Vancomycin, 343

Vancomycin-resistant *Enterococci* (VRE)
  infection, 345–347
Varicella zoster virus (VZV), 4
Vasoconstriction, 41
Vaso-occlusive crisis, 298
Ventilators, 49
Ventilatory assist, 49–50
Ventricular fibrillation, 57
Viral hepatitis serologies, 128, 130
Vital capacity (VC), 43
Vitamin B_{12}, 16
Volume-cycled ventilators, 49

W

White blood cell (WBC) count,
  118, 140, 327

Y

Yeast infections, oral, 10–12